SO-BRI-093

SCSU

JAN 2 3 2008

WITHDRAWN H.C. BULEY LIBRARY

Helping Children with Autistic Spectrum Disorders to Learn

Helping Children with Autistic Spectrum Disorders to Learn

Mary Pittman

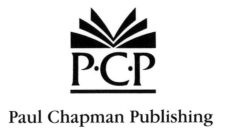

Paul Chapman Publishing

628744263
452.35

© Mary Pittman 2007

First published 2007

Apart from any fair dealing for the purposes of research or private
study, or criticism or review, as permitted under the Copyright, Designs
and Patents Act, 1988, this publication may be reproduced, stored or
transmitted in any form, or by any means, only with the prior
permission in writing of the publishers, or in the case of reprographic
reproduction, in accordance with the terms of licences issued by the
Copyright Licensing Agency. Enquiries concerning reproduction
outside those terms should be sent to the publishers.

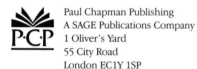

Paul Chapman Publishing
A SAGE Publications Company
1 Oliver's Yard
55 City Road
London EC1Y 1SP

SAGE Publications Inc
2455 Teller Road
Thousand Oaks, California 91320

SAGE Publications India Pvt Ltd
B 1/I1 Mohan Cooperative Industrial Area
Mathura Road, Post Bag 7
New Delhi 110 044

SAGE Publications Asia-Pacific Pte Ltd
33 Pekin Street #02-01
Far East Square
Singapore 048763

Library of Congress Control Number: 2007932988

British Library Cataloguing in Publication Data

ISBN 978-1-4129-1965-4
ISBN 978-1-4129-1966-1 (pbk)

Typeset by Pantek Arts Ltd, Maidstone, Kent
Printed in Great Britain by Cromwell Press Ltd, Trowbridge, Wiltshire
Printed on paper from sustainable resources

Dedication

To the TEACCH team in Wilmington, North Carolina, who demonstrate every good professional quality imaginable. Thank you for teaching me so much about autism and about real dedication to children and adults with autism, and their families. Your inspiration still reaches me across 3,000 miles.

Contents

List of illustrations

Acknowledgements

I feel I have struggled to be an effective teacher for my entire career. The more experience and knowledge I have gained about autism the more I realize how much there still is to learn. There are many people that I should sincerely thank for helping me in so many ways to write this book. First I want to thank all the children on the autism spectrum that I have taught, for teaching me to laugh at myself each time I got it wrong yet again! I also want to acknowledge all the teachers, teaching assistants, and parents with whom I have had the privilege to work over many years, in particular, everyone at Downham School, Plymstock, Plymouth, and everyone at Longcause School, Plympton, Plymouth. I would also like to thank a number of other people who have kept me going and ensured the completion of this book. My sincere thanks must go to: my husband, Paul Adcock, who kept the idea of writing this book alive and believed it was possible to complete it: thank you for all those 'walks and talks'; Jude Bowen and Katie Metzler, at Paul Chapman Publishing, for being patient and positive with a reluctant author; Sue Legassick, for enduring early drafts, as well as giving such useful feedback on ways of developing the book; Claire Layland and the Plymouth Communication and Interaction team for ideas and motivation. Finally I want to thank Gary Mesibov, the Director of TEACCH, for being an inspirational role model to anyone who wants to work with people who have autism and for giving me a treasured opportunity to learn both from him and from many others at TEACCH.

About the author

Mary Pittman has worked with children who have autism and other complex needs for twenty five years. In 1999 she received a National Teaching Award for her work in this field. Mary has a Master's degree in Special Education and has lectured on accredited and non-accredited training programmes for teachers and teaching assistants in the UK, as well as in other countries, such as Uganda. Mary spent seven months in 2006 working for the TEACCH programme in Wilmington, North Carolina. She works as an independent trainer and classroom adviser and is based at the Oasis Centre (Outreach, Advice, Support, Information Service) at Longcause School, Plympton, Plymouth.

About this book

My personal reasons for writing it

As a teacher with over twenty years' experience working with children on the spectrum, I have extensive knowledge of how to make mistakes with pupils who have autism. This book reflects my desire to share my own professional development with others. I have often struggled to see things from a child's perspective and allow the child to teach me where and how to make changes to my practice. In this book I am sharing strategies that I, or colleagues whom I have had the privilege to work with, have used to identify the many strengths, interests and skills that children on the autism spectrum have and how to use these to overcome areas of difficulty. Sometimes I have felt overwhelmed with all the aspects of life as a teacher and when presented with a particular child's difficulty I have forgotten to simplify the problem and remember that the child is the one who holds the answer. Simplifying the problem involves asking ourselves the question 'What do we want the child to do here?'. Once we have decided what it is that we want him to do, we can then create either a new set of circumstances or a new routine to help him respond differently, or if the child is able enough we can provide him with more information about what is expected in the situation, so that hidden knowledge is exposed and he can respond in a new way. Either way, we need to help the child make sense of what is expected in order to learn effectively.

Currently, in the UK, the National Autistic Society (NAS) is campaigning to 'make school make sense' for children on the autism spectrum. They suggest that, at present, one in 110 children have autism. Consequently, the majority of teachers will teach a child on the autism spectrum at some point during their working life. The NAS is concerned that all teachers should receive appropriate training to best support the learning needs of children on the autism spectrum. They suggest that when Sencos, teachers and other professionals understand the autism spectrum, they are better equipped to make changes to their teaching styles, the curriculum and the classroom environment.

This book has been written to support school professionals in organizing and individualizing their teaching so that children who are on the autism spectrum can become independent in using a whole range of skills for life both in school and beyond it. The book does not underestimate the many difficulties school professionals face when trying to understand and plan for students who think and learn differently. However, it does aim to simplify the problem-solving process, suggest ways of celebrating the individual strengths of children on the spectrum and provide examples of where differentiation in the way teaching is delivered can really help students on the autism spectrum to learn.

Who is the book written for?

This book recognizes the importance of real collaboration and is written to support everyone involved in educational planning for children on the autism spectrum, such as

Sencos, teachers, teaching assistants (TAs), speech therapists, parents and those in positions of care or advocacy, and of course the children themselves.

Parents can be a great source of information and insight into the way a child usually responds. When teachers and teaching assistants build reciprocal trust and communication with parents, along with other professionals, a strong team is created, and no single member of that team needs to feel under stress to know *all* the answers, or always have the right strategies to draw on. This book often refers directly to 'teachers and teaching assistants' but is written to support **all** those concerned about helping children to learn.

How to use this book

The content of the book looks at how teachers and teaching assistants can make changes to their own professional skills and knowledge, as well as the classroom environment in terms of timetable information, working systems, clear tasks and curriculum balance as well as contributing towards whole-school support systems in order that each student on the autism spectrum has an effective education programme.

The book considers examples of practice in a variety of school settings and also provides case study examples of children who are functioning at a variety of levels in terms of their cognitive abilities and their degree of autism. The reader can therefore gain a good overall understanding of autism and the issues which arise in teaching and learning across the spectrum, but can also focus and apply sections of the book which are specific to their own professional, student or setting needs.

Each chapter presents subheadings to show the key areas being covered in the chapter. Some of the main sections have interactive exercises within them to help readers consider their own thoughts, or which can be used by Sencos, or others involved in providing professional development, in understanding and teaching children with autism. A brief outline of the chapters is given below.

1 Interpreting autism as a triad of opportunity

Chapter 1 provides an overview of the three key areas of difficulty which define autism, known as the triad of impairment. The chapter looks at the range of responses that children present, so as to provide teachers and teaching assistants with a wider framework for understanding the spectrum. The chapter sets the scene and encourages us to see our role as a dual interpreter, firstly translating autism for colleagues and then interpreting social cues for children on the autism spectrum. It also focuses on understanding each individual child's unique presentation of autism. Readers can use the content of this chapter to consider how, by modifying their own interactions and communication when teaching, they can help children with autism to feel more relaxed and ready to learn. The chapter suggests that professionals interpret the triad of impairment as a triad of opportunity, using an understanding of autism to interact and teach more effectively.

2 The autism-friendly professional

This chapter focuses on the professionals who work with children on the autism spectrum. It looks at how a knowledge of autism, and of individual differences in the presentation of autism, can enable readers to be empathetic and insightful professionals. The chapter considers the expectations professionals have of themselves and those that students and parents may have of them. Readers can use this chapter to reflect on the roles they play in supporting and teaching children on the autism spectrum. The chapter considers the difficulties, dilemmas and rewards of these roles. The chapter encourages us to evaluate our own development as professionals who understand autism and its implications for teaching and learning. Readers can also use the chapter to reflect on the support mechanisms they may need to decrease their own stress and focus on enabling children on the autism spectrum to learn.

3 Making sense of changes and transitions

Everyone experiences changes occurring in their daily lives on a large or small scale. Consequently we all recognize that 'changes' can happen in a number of forms and demand different responses from us.

This chapter considers in depth one particular area of difficulty for children on the autism spectrum, understanding and accepting changes in daily routines and situations. This chapter considers how 'a change is only a change' if you recognize it as such and discusses the complexities of individual responses to 'change', which can cause real stress for children on the autism spectrum. Strategies are suggested for helping children to perceive change differently, or understand and accept change.

4 Structuring a meaningful classroom

'Structuring a meaningful classroom' considers what we mean by structured teaching and how this approach can help to make the classroom make sense. It considers how teachers and teaching assistants can learn most from observing and listening to each individual about what helps him learn. Readers can use this chapter to focus on where and how they can make small adjustments to differentiate learning, clarify expectations and organize the classroom day. Ways of using timetables and working systems can give predictability to students and also be used to teach flexibility and independence.

5 Behaviour; simplifying the problem-solving process

This chapter considers how some children on the autism spectrum communicate their frustrations through their behaviour. It focuses on the ways in which teachers and TAs can support themselves and other colleagues through the problem-solving process and can use simple questions to try and formulate a clear strategy for resolving challenging behaviour. The chapter considers how stress manifests itself through behaviour and how this can affect both pupils on the autism spectrum and those that work with them. The chapter suggests the use of an approach referred to as SPACE (Stress, Prevention, Action, Calming Environments and Extras) as a means of distancing both the pupil and the staff from the challenging behaviour.

6 Frequently asked questions

Chapter 6 considers some of the questions often asked by Sencos, teachers and teaching assistants in primary, secondary and special schools. Some are dealt with as generic issues, while other questions are context-specific, with particular reference to primary, secondary and special school settings. They address the needs of children who are experiencing autism at different levels of severity, and with or without additional learning difficulties. Readers can use this chapter to revisit or clarify information, focus on specific areas, or broaden their knowledge and insights by reading the questions, answers and examples which are different from their own.

How you can interact with the book

The book provides some experiential exercises that can be used to give insights into the difficulties faced by students who are on the spectrum. These experiential exercises in no way suggest that we can truly understand and feel what it is like to be on the autism spectrum. However, some exercises of this nature may help us gain insight into one or two of the areas of difficulty and provide us with renewed empathy.

The book also provides some case studies which demonstrate successful practice along with exercises which ask us to reflect upon our own practice. These exercises aim to help teachers and teaching assistants (TAs) to strengthen their observation, assessment and strategy implementation skills.

In addition, the book provides planning exercises to apply to the classroom or school situation, which may help professionals be as proactive in preventing difficulties arising as they also need to be in reacting to new challenges which a child on the autism spectrum may present.

I strongly believe that children on the autism spectrum learn most effectively from visual information. To illustrate the use of visual tools when teaching children on the autism spectrum a number of visual images, photographs, and diagrams are used in this book to support the text.

The word 'autism' literally means 'self state', which immediately tells us that anyone who has this disability will have difficulty establishing a clear concept of themselves, which in turn leads to a lack of understanding of other people. It makes sense when considering the meaning of autism that relating to others, interacting socially and a whole array of communication and thinking skills which children usually acquire are likely to be different or difficult for children who are diagnosed as on the autism spectrum.

When referring to children on the autism spectrum, this book uses the word 'spectrum' to include the full range of children who have an Autistic Spectrum Disorder (ASD). When using phrases such as 'children on the autism spectrum' the book is referring to those with mild, moderate or severe autism, children with Asperger's syndrome or high-functioning autism (HFA) and pupils who have autism with or without learning difficulties or co-occurring difficulties. The terms 'child' and 'pupil' will be used interchangeably as appropriate and the pronoun 'he' has been selected for use rather than 'she' when generally referring to a child purely to provide continuity, ease of reading and reference. Throughout the book there are composite case studies and comments which reflect a wide range of school contexts and experience across the autism spectrum.

Interpreting Autism as a Triad of Opportunity

People on the autism spectrum have difficulties in three areas, social interaction, communication and flexible and imaginative thinking, referred to by Lorna Wing (1996) as the triad of impairment. There has been a lot of very thorough and helpful information written about the three key areas of difficulty which define autism. This chapter provides an overview of the characteristics of autism and portrays some of the numerous ways in which children on the spectrum present their unique autism profile.

This chapter looks at the following:

- What do we mean by the autism spectrum and the three key areas of difficulty that define autism?

- How do we see individuals with autism behaving across the spectrum?

- How can we create teaching and learning opportunities from our knowledge and understanding of autism?

This chapter explores the three key areas of difficulty for children on the autism spectrum and the range of responses that individual pupils present. The chapter provides professional development activities to enable us to reflect upon our understanding of autism and consider how we can match our teaching approach to each child's unique presentation of autism. The chapter challenges us to think creatively about how we can make the 'triad of impairment' a 'triad of opportunity' by using our knowledge of autism to plan effective teaching and learning opportunities.

To help us understand and empathize with children on the autism spectrum this chapter asks us to reflect on some of our own experiences and behaviours, which sometimes give us insights into how individuals with autism may respond. However, it is important not to trivialize the impact of autism through our own insights into one or two of the behaviours that we can personally identify with. The chapter considers the social interaction skills, communication skills and the flexible imaginative thinking skills which most of us can access easily without much conscious thought, in an effort to try and appreciate how complicated apparently simple interactions and communications are, if like children on the autism spectrum we do not possess such skills. The chapter also highlights that, in addition to the three specific areas of difficulty, the interrelationship of these areas further complicates the way each person on the spectrum thinks, acts and understands the world around him.

What do we mean by autism and the autism spectrum?

Autism is a communication difficulty, which makes it difficult for children on the autism spectrum to:

- Listen and relate to others.
- Recognize and understand the meaning of facial expressions, gestures, body language and the emotions that they signify.
- Interpret social signals, and understand what others want from you.
- Work out what others are saying.
- Imagine what to do in unfamiliar situations.
- Be clear about fact and fantasy.
- Think about things from the perspective of others.
- Think flexibly and accept changes.

Autism is a neurological developmental disability which, say Mesibov, *et al.* (2004), 'affects the ways that individuals, think, eat, dress, work, spend leisure time, understand their world, communicate, etc'. Mesibov *et al.* (2004) provide a very useful analogy in that autism is seen to some degree to be a 'culture'. Although they recognize that autism is not in actuality a culture, the predictable patterns of thinking and behaviour that people with autism share provide a clear commonality. As autism is a spectrum there are numerous factors which contribute to the uniqueness of each individual with autism. The term 'spectrum' reminds us to respect the individuality of each person with autism. This includes understanding the mild, moderate or severe degree of their autism, recognizing the cognitive abilities of each person with it, and setting this alongside a whole range of other distinct factors including particular skills, interests, age, personality, etc.

Throughout this book, the phrase 'children on the autism spectrum' is used to refer to **all** children with an Autistic Spectrum Disorder (ASD). This includes children with Aspergers Syndrome, high functioning autism (HFA), as well as pupils who have autism with or without learning difficulties or co-occurring difficulties, at varying degrees from mild to severe.

Introducing the triad of impairment

This chapter focuses on exploring, across the spectrum, the range of behaviours which characterize autism, within each area of the triad of impairment: social interaction, language and communication and inflexibility of thought and impairment in imagination. However, before doing so the chapter asks us to reflect upon the usual range of responses that neuro-typical people demonstrate in terms of these three areas, before continuing to explore the difficulties which children and adults on the autism spectrum have in relation to these areas of development.

Each area of the triad of impairment will be considered in turn. Firstly the way autism affects how a person understands and uses interaction skills as a means of building relationships with others and making social judgements will be discussed. Secondly, how autism affects the way a person processes and uses language along with the whole range of non-verbal communication skills such as gestures, facial and body language. Thirdly there will be a focus on how autism affects a person's perception of what is happening and limits their range of imaginative responses.

Each area of the triad of impairment causes real difficulties in itself, and many of the behaviours that we see in autism can be exhibited by children with a whole range of other learning differences. For a child to be diagnosed as being on the autism spectrum, he must show characteristics from each of the three key areas of difficulty. The interrelationship of the features from all the areas results in a person being unable to understand the often covert and subtle messages or meanings that guide our usual social communications and behaviour in relation to our age, gender, culture and other factors. Each person with autism will vary in the extent to which they are affected and the cognitive skills they have to enable them to learn coping mechanisms or social understanding.

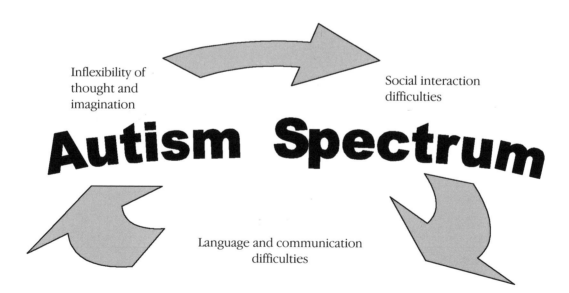

Inflexibility of thought and imagination

Social interaction difficulties

Language and communication difficulties

Figure I The triad of impairment comprising the spectrum of autism

The word 'spectrum' helps us to understand that there are a variety of factors affecting the unique presentations of autism that each child displays. A primary factor is the severity of the autism itself. Children can be affected by autism in a mild, moderate or severe way and may additionally have other learning differences contributing to their own individual autism and learning profile.

It can be helpful for teachers and teaching assistants to be able to identify the full range of behaviours that they may see different pupils on the autism spectrum exhibiting, understanding that they arise from features within the same three key areas of difficulty. This enables us to recognize how the triad of impairment is impacting on each individual child and how important it is to our teaching approach that we plan successful learning activities by taking account of the individual autism characteristics, cognitive abilities and personalities of children on the spectrum. Teachers and TAs can really benefit from a full 'spectrum' knowledge.

Before considering how people on the autism spectrum may interact, communicate and think it is important to consider how most of us usually operate within these areas. By doing this we can gain insights into the very skills, behaviours and understanding that children on the autism spectrum do not acquire easily. Many of these interpersonal skills are used by most of us without much conscious thought and these are often the very skills which children on the autism spectrum find difficult to understand or use.

How do we see individuals with autism behaving across the spectrum? Let's look at the triad of impairment – social interaction; language and communication; mental inflexibility – more closely.

Social interaction

For most people, interacting is part of our everyday experience. Most people are able to initiate interaction, position themselves in relation to others in terms of personal space, use and read eye contact, facial expressions and gestures to clarify and add meaning to their spoken communication. There are some variations in how effective and perceptive people generally are in social settings but on the whole people tend to share an understanding of non-verbal clues. Children usually learn with indirect teaching, experience and sometimes direct explanation about where and how to read and use a range of signals and acquire a knowledge of developmentally appropriate social conduct. As children grow older and mature they often update their knowledge of social expectations, whereas children on the autism spectrum struggle with understanding or using social interaction skills and then struggle with how they update and change according to their age or the circumstances they find themselves in. This often leaves them misunderstood and isolated.

In order for us to really consider the skills involved in social interaction the staff training activity on the next page may be a helpful starting point. This activity highlights how important an understanding of personal space, eye contact, facial signals and body language are to our interactive communication with others and how these intertwine with what we hear in conversation or say as part of our back-and-forth reciprocal communication with others.

Staff training activity

UNDERSTANDING SOCIAL INTERACTION SKILLS AND DIFFICULTIES

The activity could be used as an ice-breaker to a training session or to promote staff discussion. The exercise tries to give us insight into the hidden barrier to learning which social interaction difficulties present for children on the autism spectrum.

Ask staff to break into pairs and spend three to five minutes interacting with each other

Suggest the staff find someone that they do not usually spend much time with or do not know well and spend some time talking with them about what questions they have about autism or what difficulties they would like to overcome as they work with a particular child, or spend some time generally getting to know a little about the other person's role/work, etc. Encourage enough time for people to enjoy the interaction and have time to be fully involved in it but do not let this experience become too long and unfocused.

Observe the interactions

Observe so that in the discussion about interaction skills you can report on what you saw to help illustrate points. Or stop people where they are standing and sitting and discuss what they are doing in terms of body position, *eye contact, use of gestures, facial expression, ways of communicating points*, etc.

Ask for feedback on the skills used by using prompt questions such as:

- How did you position yourself for this social interaction and communication? (*Body position and recognition of appropriate space*)
- How did you let the other person know you were listening to them and interested in what they had to say? (*Eye contact, nodding, smiling*)
- How did the other person show you that they were connecting to what you were saying and meaning? (*Turn taking in the conversation*)
- How did you know the other person was empathetic and interested in what you were saying? (*Facial signals, emotional balance, e.g. laughed or was serious to mirror what was being conveyed, etc.*)

Review what a person on the autism spectrum might behave like in an interaction situation. Ask staff to consider:

- If someone is unable to make accurate guesses about what people are thinking or feeling, and is unable to read their facial expressions, how might they act or appear to someone trying to interact with them?
- If someone is unable to use eye contact correctly, or understand the eye contact signals from someone else, how might they appear to a person trying to interact with them?
- If someone is unable to adjust their emotional reactions to mirror another person, how might they appear to a person trying to interact with them?
- If someone is unable to select relevant social clues and signals, how might they appear to a person trying to interact with them?

After the 'social interaction' focus of the exercise is explored any questions and difficulties that staff raised during their discussions, in other words the content of their discussions, could be noted and shared or clarified during further training.

In considering social interaction skills, eye contact with another person usually gives us vital information and we use it to give information too. Eye contact is a sign we are listening to someone, that there is shared attention, that we have a social connection with another person. We use our eyes to give other non-verbal messages too, that we agree with a person, or need clarification. We also know how to read these same eye contact messages from others.

We read other facial signals too and link them with the emotions that people are feeling. We know the meaning of a frown, a smile, etc. We know that when we see someone raise their eyes we may read that they are surprised or not sure they agree on that point.

As part of our emotional empathy and social understanding we position ourselves and use our body position and adjust those positions as is helpful to an interaction and as the formality or informality of the situation demands. Gestures are also used to emphasize points or substitute words when we are unclear how to put things.

To a person who is on the autism spectrum these actions do not naturally provide the same clues or have the same meaning and, coupled with difficulties processing verbal information, are part of their confusion about what is expected of them rather than supportive and clarifying.

What range of social interaction responses can we expect to see from a child on the autism spectrum?

From considering the reactions that we usually expect in terms of social interaction it is important to then focus on the range of interactive behaviours that we might observe children or adults on the autism spectrum using. Some social interaction behaviours are usual at one age and not another, some social interaction behaviours could be considered at one developmental age and not another. Therefore any unusual reactions that we observe in the area of social interaction, or any other area, needs to be observed and measured in relation to the child's age and his developmental learning level.

Eye contact and facial signals

Many adults with autism explain that using eye contact or looking at others when interacting may not provide the useful clues and meaning that it does for those of us not on the autism spectrum. Opportunities to listen to adults who are on the autism spectrum, give us the most useful insights into what eye contact or other facial signals might mean or not mean to them.

People kept saying just look at me when I'm talking to you. I wanted to say when I look at your face I can't hear what you're saying.
(Adult with autism)

It is important to look at people when you talk to them. My mum had to tell me that. I didn't know that other people expected me to look at them.
(Adult with autism)

Sometimes people suggest that children and adults who are on the autism spectrum do not make eye contact at all. In reality is it more common to notice that eye contact is being used in unusual or more limited ways than would usually be the case. Each individual on the autism spectrum will show his own individual style and level of eye contact and these may or may not differ in relation to factors such as familiarity, level of stress, level of interest, etc.

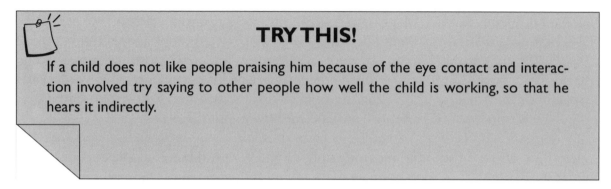

TRY THIS!

If a child does not like people praising him because of the eye contact and interaction involved try saying to other people how well the child is working, so that he hears it indirectly.

Each individual person on the autism spectrum will use and understand the meaning of eye contact differently. Eye contact may be fleeting, peripheral, intense and without regard for personal space, or it may be a sustained gaze but looking beyond or even through people. Sometimes children on the spectrum will use a range of different kinds of eye contact, depending upon the situation. When a child is feeling very relaxed, his eye contact response may vary. He may look at someone more frequently or in a more usual way.

TRY THIS!

During lessons if a child does not look at the teacher while they are talking and giving information about the lesson, check and see whether the child listens better when he is focused on holding or squeezing something in his hand, e.g. a stress ball. If the child can answer questions or knows what he has been asked to do this might help him listen more effectively rather than looking directly at the teacher or TA.

Pupils with ASD also have difficulties reading other facial expressions. They also find gestures which we use to support or substitute for language hard to understand. For example, sometimes we frown, or shake our head, and the child is unable to read these signals. It is important therefore to remember that children may find it hard to follow subtle signals given by school staff to try and direct or redirect them in the classroom. They may even be amused by certain facial expressions that are not meant to be amusing.

TRY THIS!

If a pupil is ready to learn the meaning of facial expressions, as well as teaching the more obvious and distinctive ones – happy, sad, angry, etc. – try also to teach what faces look like when the person is not conveying a major emotion, just a thinking or resting face.

Imitation

We often in one-to-one interactions mirror and imitate what others are expressing in terms of emotional and social references. We also in new social situations watch to see what we should do and copy the actions of others if things are not familiar to us. Children and adults on the autism spectrum may display a range of differences in the way they use imitation skills. For example, they may not notice what others are doing or may not be able to select which actions are relevant to imitate. Some people on the autism spectrum may also display differences in the way they mirror someone else in a situation, and some people may not notice that an adjustment would be appropriate in that situation.

Pupils on the autism spectrum will have a variety of differences in the way they imitate others and use it as a skill to learn. It is helpful to observe the way a pupil you work with copies or does not copy his peers or learns by an adult demonstrating what to do. Consider the following differences in social imitation skills that you might observe in pupils on the spectrum.

Some pupils may:

- Be unaware of what other children and adults around them are doing.

- Imitate one particular pupil only, someone who he regularly sits with, for example.

- Imitate what others do but without understanding why. Jake, a Year 7 boy, copied another student in how to use the school canteen. He imitated not only the process of what to do in terms of the sequence of collecting his meal but also imitated his peer in choosing the same lunch even though he disliked the food choices and could not eat it.

- Not be able to select the most appropriate peer to imitate and may choose the wrong role model.

- Be unable to generalize what has been imitated in a specific situation into another situation.

Reading 'between the lines'

Most people have learnt that there are 'hidden' rules which we need to be aware of in all social situations that we find ourselves in. We have learnt through each stage of our growing-up process that we often need to adjust our behaviours and make social judgements based on who we are with and what would be appropriate in each situation. Children and adults on the autism spectrum have real difficulties understanding what the social expectations are in different contexts. In the context of school and the classroom, so many situations depend upon a child realizing what is expected and what the 'hidden' curriculum is expecting of them.

CASE STUDY: KELLY

Kelly, a pupil with autism and moderate learning difficulties, continually shouted out comments or answers to questions in the classroom. She had been told on numerous occasions to put her hand up if she wanted to say something or ask a question. Sometimes she would put her hand up quickly then put it down and continue to shout out and over other pupils.

What might staff think the behaviour was about?
Initially staff might feel that Kelly was ignoring the classroom rule to put her hand up and was refusing to listen and comply.

What else could it be?
Kelly did seem to be trying to respond and did, albeit very quickly, put her hand in the air. Perhaps she did not understand the procedure of putting your hand up, keeping it there and waiting for someone to ask you to speak, because these were implied rather than stated in the instruction to 'put your hand up'.

How did Kelly's autism affect her behaviour?
Kelly was very literal in how she interpreted what was said to her. She was also unable to 'read between the lines' of any information not made totally explicit to her. This resulted in her not being able to do the right thing, even when staff felt they had directed her to do so by telling her to 'put her hand up'.

What did staff do to help Kelly?
The staff wrote down and explained to Kelly what she needed to do so that she could fully understand each step of raising her hand, keeping it in the air and waiting to be asked her answer or what she wanted to say. This time Kelly could use her literal interpretation skills, as the steps provided were clear enough to be helpful rather than unhelpful and she did not need to 'read between the lines', which was one of her major difficulties.

Later staff also wrote an explanation of what she needed to do if another child was chosen to answer.

In school, pupils on the spectrum may have greater difficulty than other students in understanding that different teachers or teaching assistants may have differences in what they expect in terms of the working environment. Each year group, class or department may have different rules, routines and implicit expectations. For a child on the spectrum implicit expectations will often need to be made explicit, with some pupils also benefiting from clear and logical explanations which give reasons why it is helpful if they concentrate, behave and work in a particular way. Some pupils do understand the specific social or learning rules for a particular situation but they may be unable to generalize them in other classes or situations or may have difficulty recognizing where they do not need to be adhered to, or are unnecessary. Either way, misunderstandings can easily arise when a child on the autism spectrum is unclear, unable to generalize or over-zealous with any hidden rules that require him to read between the lines.

Understanding emotions

People on the autism spectrum find it hard to read the emotional signals that other people present facially when interacting. They can also be less animated in their facial expressions or body language. Some children and adults on the autism spectrum may not be able to show facially how they are feeling, and this in itself can cause difficulties in terms of other people reading signals about changes to the person's mood, or tolerance, and not therefore having available the usual signals. Children may also find it hard to predict what others may think or feel in situations.

Shifting attention

Shifting attention requires that children stop and move their attention from one subject being talked about to another or from one activity being carried out to another, and particularly from one person to another. Often in the classroom we ask pupils to stop for a moment, we add in information and then expect them to return to concentrating on their work. For children with autism who have difficulties becoming engaged in their learning, and also difficulties disengaging once they are engaged, these seemingly small parts of classroom life can be more complex than we realize.

Language and communication

It is as usual for children to developmentally acquire interaction skills and social understanding as it is with other areas of development such as language and communication. Language and communication is the second area of the triad of impairment and involves how a child processes and understands language as well as how he uses language expressively.

Spoken language is a usual mode of communication for most children and adults and an understanding of the way we acquire the skill can, as with social interaction skills, help us to gain insights into the developmental level that a child is both responding to and using in spoken language.

What language and communication behaviours might children on the autism spectrum display?

Children on the autism spectrum usually have a selection of receptive and expressive language differences. Receptively there may be processing and comprehension difficulties to varying degrees. Expressively there will be difficulties with using language with communicative intent to varying degrees.

TRY THIS!

■ Always use the **name** of the child/student and give clear precise instructions.

■ If repeating a specific and well constructed instruction, **try using the same words again** rather than rewording it, so the child only has to reprocess part of the instruction again.

In addition children on the autism spectrum may not understand or use the social communication features of language in terms of tone, volume, pitch, or understanding what clues these usually give us when attaching meaning to the words being used.

Children who have high functioning autism or Asperger's syndrome may use formal or adult language and may well use excessive details when describing what has happened.

Literal interpretation

Children on the autism spectrum who can process language and understand it may still have problems in that their interpretation of what they hear said may be very literal and therefore confusing in terms of the literal images it visually conveys to the children. To interpret literally means to understand the words exactly and factually rather than recognizing any associated meanings or actions.

Metaphors, sarcasm, questions requesting a reply through action or implication, all require an understanding of associated social meanings which children on the autism spectrum find particularly difficult.

Joel, a secondary school student, responded literally when his teacher told him, 'It's time you pulled your socks up, young man,' which resulted in his peers laughing and the student on the autism spectrum appearing to be behaving badly when in fact he was pulling his socks up because he was taking his teacher's comment literally. Nathan, a primary pupil, was very upset when he heard people saying, 'It's raining cats and dogs,' by covering his ears and shouting, 'It's not true, it's not true.'

Sometimes interpreting literally can mean that the pupil is not able to understand that what appears like a question is really an instruction. For example, if a pupil is asked, 'Sue, can you open the window?' Sue might answer, 'Yes, I can,' and not do what she was asked because she was unaware that the question was really a request for action.

Literal interpretation can extend to the written as well as the spoken word, so when writing instructions for pupils who can read them, we need to ensure that we have been clear and specific and not expect pupils on the autism spectrum to 'read between the lines'.

Kevin, for example, was following written instructions in a food technology lesson when he read, 'Sprinkle flour on the worktop and roll the pastry.' Kevin proceeded to sprinkle flour on the worktop and then to put a knife along the edge of the worktop as if trying to damage it. When asked what he was doing he explained that he had to get the worktop up to roll his pastry, He immediately understood when we wrote the line again so that it said 'Sprinkle flour on the worktop, then, using a rolling pin, roll out the pastry.'

Try using the exercise 'Making classroom language clear', on page 16, to help you clarify some spoken or written instructions which you might use in your classroom.

Echolalia

Some children or adults on the autism spectrum display echolalia, whereby they repeat what they have heard. Children can be observed using immediate echolalia or delayed echolalia or both.

If you ask a child, 'Do you want a drink?' they may use immediate echolalia and:

- repeat back the last word, e.g. 'drink'.

- repeat back part of the phrase, e.g. 'want a drink'.

- repeat back the whole sentence, 'Do you want a drink?'.

If a child quotes from videos or DVDs, or repeats information heard some time ago, this might be delayed echolalia.

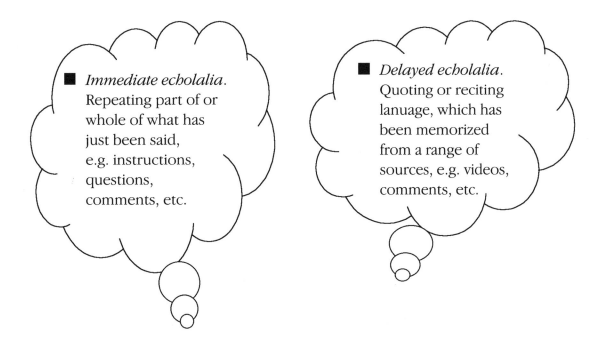

- *Immediate echolalia*. Repeating part of or whole of what has just been said, e.g. instructions, questions, comments, etc.

- *Delayed echolalia*. Quoting or reciting lanuage, which has been memorized from a range of sources, e.g. videos, comments, etc.

MAKING CLASSROOM LANGUAGE CLEAR

Using the examples below write a brief explanation of what some classroom instructions really mean so that a pupil on the autism spectrum could read and understand more definitely what they need to do:

- When a teacher says, 'Line up,' the teacher really means: ....

    ....

    ....

    ....

- When a teacher asks you to put your hand up if you want to speak this means put

    your hand up and ....

- Some teachers say, 'Listen up, everyone,' others say .... Both mean the

    same thing. They mean that ....

If you are working with pupils who cannot read or follow more complex explanations, consider these classroom instructions and how you might make them more understandable using additional cues, e.g. visual or auditory, practising skills, using consistent language, etc.

Echolalia helps us to see that a child is processing language. There are a number of interesting theories about the reasons for and functions of echolalia and it is worth considering how it is being used by a pupil who displays it.

Some children may use their 'video-speak' echolalia in situations as a way of relating to what is happening. Jessica loved Disney videos and would often entertain herself by repeating sections of a video. Sometimes she would use this sort of language in real situations too. If she or another child was upset for any reason, and in tears, she would respond by saying, 'The beautiful princess was so very sad, the tears ran down her cheeks.'

Children on the autism spectrum have different reasons for using immediate or delayed echolalia. In some situations children with more severe autism who have limited verbal abilities may use a phrase to initiate contact, to help them process language, to make a request or to just have fun. Alternatively they may express a phrase repeatedly with an anxious tone to express confusion and distress. For pupils with autism and severe learning difficulties this can sometimes be one of the few ways they can express their frustrations or anxieties. Lucy, a student with severe autism and severe learning difficulties who attended a special school, would use the phrase 'Ice cream? Maybe later,' using a phrase that she had heard others use to her. Depending on her tone of voice and the situation she was using it in, the staff worked out whether she was anxious or making a request or wanting to say hello to them.

Understanding or using emphasis

Some children and adults may have real differences in interpreting a change in emphasis in the way one word in a sentence is said. The following activity can be carried out for self-reflection or as staff development exercises which help to develop awareness and understanding of some of the language differences which children or adults on the autism spectrum may experience.

EXERCISE

Changing emphasis changes meaning

Read out loud the following sentence. Vocally emphasize the underlined word and each time notice how the change in emphasis changes the meaning of the sentence.

- I didn't say he was speaking to me.
- I didn't say he was speaking to me.
- I didn't say he was speaking to me.
- I didn't say he was speaking to me.
- I didn't say he was speaking to me.
- I didn't say he was speaking to me.

Children on the autism spectrum may find it difficult to use the pronouns 'I' and 'you' in the correct places and or may substitute others for them. Some children use their name rather than the pronoun 'I', e.g. 'Katie wants cake.' Other children may use the questions or phrases they have heard others say to them and use them to make their own requests, e.g. 'Do you want a drink, do you?'

Some children find it hard to understand or use melody, intonation, vocal tone, volume adjustments variation in pitch, stress and rhythm to indicate emotions or social appropriateness.

Children or adults on the autism spectrum may be unable to initiate conversation, or may use a set phrase as their method of doing this. Some children may use a phrase such as 'Guess what.' to gain the attention of someone or start a conversation. Some children do not know how to start a conversation, or what questions they could ask others to start a conversation.

TRY THIS!

- As children on the autism spectrum have difficulties processing questions and then formulating their reply try to **reduce questions** and instead **use statements** to gain an answer. Rather than ask 'What is the man doing in the picture?' try saying 'The man in the picture is ....' and pausing for a reply.

Inflexible thought and imagination

Difficulties with flexible and imaginative thinking can mean that a child on the autism spectrum has difficulties with:

- Understanding and accepting changes to their usual routines or circumstances.

- Being creative in play or other imaginative activities.

- Establishing a clear concept of finish or completion to activities.

Change

As inflexibility of thought is one of the three major areas of difficulty for children with autism it is no surprise that children on the spectrum are likely to display a range of differences in the ways they understand and are affected by changes that we make to their day, or that just happen in day-to-day life.

Children on the autism spectrum can feel under stress when faced with changes which require them to be flexible in thinking, and imagination, and require them to make a new response.

EXERCISE

School: a changing context

In school as in any context there are likely to be a number of changes which children on the autism spectrum will need to negotiate at some time. As a reflection activity or a staff development activity consider where and when and how these changes occur:

■ Changes in the sequence of lessons.

■ Changes in classroom routines.

■ Changes in the classroom environment.

■ Starting in a new class.

■ Changing schools.

■ School holidays and restarting back at school.

Consider which of the above areas a pupil you work with has difficulties with.

Play

Children on the autism spectrum find it hard to play in the usual imaginative ways. As with all other aspects of autism, there are a range of ways in which this may be displayed, such as:

■ Toys used to make an organized pattern rather than to be creative or symbolic.

■ A routine of elaborate play actions but carried out repetitively with all toys.

■ Little contact with objects, or sensory and based in the earliest levels of development.

TRY THIS!

If a young child with autism does not copy your actions in a play situation, and does not interact very much with objects but does do some repetative actions, e.g. tapping, then **try copying his actions** instead.

Leroy, a pupil in a foundation stage class, avoided using the writing and drawing activity tables in his classroom. Whenever his TA tried to encourage him to make marks of any kind on paper he showed no interest and if she tried encouraging him by putting her hand over his he resisted. The only thing he did was tap the pencils or pens being used.

His TA sat opposite him with a large piece of paper and some pens and copied what he did. After tapping for a short while and watching his TA tapping, he suddenly made a mark on the paper and looked at his TA's hand to see if she copied him. Using this method Leroy's resistance to using pens and pencils was overcome and he began to enjoy drawing shapes and writing letters.

Special interests

Children on the autism spectrum often have special interests which may be in the form of a particular action, activity or subject to talk about. Often these special interests can be useful for relaxing or motivating children. When children can enjoy these interests and can easily be diverted from them and back on to directed tasks they can be very useful and usable. If a child has a range of interests this can be useful: where one of them becomes obsessional others can be substituted. However, when a child becomes very intense about his special interest and fixed upon it to the exclusion of other areas then the special interest may be becoming an obsession. Special interests often tend to increase to obsession level when the person on the autism spectrum is feeling under stress.

Once a special interest has become an obsession it is likely to require negotiated management to ensure that it is useful rather than preventing learning.

Some pupils feel under stress when the time they are allocated in school to do their special interest is limited and it may even become stressful rather than helpful to have that time. Sometimes creating books about a child's unusual and not easily usable special interest can help. If, for example, a child has an interest in a particular place, or the computer, or a Playstation game, or an activity which is not easily or regularly accessible, then making books about that interest and giving him some time to look at them can also be a good substitute.

CASE STUDY: RAJINDER

For Rajinder, a fourteen-year-old student who attended a special school, using the computer and any aspect of ICT was a special interest. For several weeks he worked hard to earn tokens to gain time to use the computer at the end of the school day for fifteen minutes three days a week. Gradually he began to ask over and over again, had he been good, when was he going to use the computer, could he print out pictures, or play certain games, and his queries about using it became very demanding and began distracting him from his work.

What might staff think the behaviour was about?

Initially staff felt that Rajinder was demanding more and more talk time about the computer and even when told when he could use it he continued to keep asking. As soon as he had his fifteen minutes on it he would ask when the next time was.

What else could it be?

When staff discussed the situation they realized that on the days he did not have the computer but did reading his books at the end of the day, he was much calmer and did not ask about the computer. This implied that he knew which days he was having it, so that was not the issue he was finding hard.

How did Rajinder's autism affect his behaviour?

Rajinder's constant asking was as much a stress for him as it became for the staff. Rajinder was unable to stop thinking about when his time on the computer would be that day, and his keenness to have that time seemed to make him anxious rather than relaxed. The time he spent on the computer was also quite short and it was not easy for him to feel satisfied with what he could achieve.

What could staff do to help Rajinder?

It was decided to tell Rajinder at the end of the week that the following week he would have reading time at the end of each day instead of computer leisure time. A paper was typed out with symbols and photographs, explaining clearly what would start happening the following week. Time was negotiated with his parents at weekends for him to use his home computer for leisure and to keep his school use work-related. When Rajinder initially read about this and had it explained, he accepted it, but was not entirely happy about the change of plan. However, when he came to school the next week he was much happier and much less stressed, as he now knew what he would do each day to finish his day, and he knew when he could use the computer for his leisure and have more definite time to enjoy it fully.

It is important to notice if a special interest is becoming stressful rather than restful and motivating in children with autism.

Phobias

Some people on the autism spectrum encounter specific and extreme fears or phobias which may be based upon their imaginative difficulties in understanding fact and fantasy. For some children phobias are based on the unpredictable response of the object or thing which they are afraid of.

One secondary school Year 7 student suffered from extreme fear of dogs. One of the problems that the staff at school experienced with this student was his erratic moods at the start of the school day. Sometimes he was calm and quite focused, at other times very strained and lacking concentration. There appeared to be no particular pattern to this behaviour. However, in speaking to his parent it transpired that when they walked to school, if they saw a dog it meant that they had to turn round and walk another way, which often meant they were late and the student started the day not feeling calm or ready to work.

Pupils who have phobias are very conscious of them and have a heightened awareness in relation to the object of the phobia. One primary-age pupil, who had an extreme anxiety about balloons, could always see a balloon at a considerable distance.

Some students experience phobias that develop associations, for example children who develop anxieties about hay because it is linked with animals.

Some children need information that they can read and so develop an understanding of the thing which is causing them to be fearful. However, some children who may have a limited understanding may require a careful programme that helps to desensitize them.

Always seek help and permission from the child's parents to work on any anxiety or fear which a pupil is experiencing. Also request support and guidance from relevant professionals to ensure that any strategies or programmes are appropriate. Consult parents, psychologists, teachers from the Communication and Interaction team, before attempting to address any major anxiety areas.

For children on the autism spectrum who can read and understand information it is useful to review practical resources for such children which provide examples of how to write the facts or provide options as to what the child can do in situations which help them cope.

With children who cannot understand written information, observe at what level they are comfortable with their fear. This may involve showing the child pictures, or providing a recording of sounds or symbolic representations of the object of his fear. Identify where the child shows mild anxiety and focus on this – on letting the child see, hear or experience it. Ensure that you follow this short exposure time with time doing something very relaxing and enjoyable.

Special objects

Some young or developmentally young children with autism want to carry an object around with them. Some objects are small and easy to carry, and the child is able to trade them, or put them in a set place, while doing other things, and then have them back afterwards. When teaching a child to trade an object that is important to him, it can help to use a transparent container with a lid, to put it in, so that he can still see it is available to use, have back, after an activity. With some children who have very severe autism objects can feel vital and sensitive handling is needed to modify their use within acceptable levels.

Transition

A transition is about the finishing of one activity or situation and the beginning of another one. A child has difficulties with transitioning from one activity to another, one place to another because of difficulties with being able to:

- Understand when things are finished.
- Predict what is next.
- Have time to adjust to stopping or starting.
- Understand any lack of structure in the transition period.

Some of the range of reactions that may be observed could be: upset, reluctance or slowness to finish one activity, taking time to pack up as if giving the self time to come to terms with the need to change over activities.

Children on the autism spectrum have a strong visual memory for what they experience, see or read and this is a very valuable strength. However, there are times when this visual strength can be an overactive method of prediction for children on the autism spectrum. Therefore they memorize what they believe the sequence of events will be and they can be upset when things do not happen in that way and may try to insist on it happening as they visually have memorised it. They may experience real distress and a feeling that they cannot continue with anything else because they must go through with what they have started to do.

Prompt-dependence issues

Some children on the autistic spectrum can become prompt-dependent, waiting for verbal direction. For example, Molly was a young child who often came out of the toilet without flushing it.

Most people instructed her to 'flush' and she would go back in and do so. It was not long before she was coming out of the bathroom and waiting. Sometimes she would say over and over, 'flush, flush,' until she was told, 'Yes, go and flush.' This instruction became part of the toileting routine.

Some children may be much less independent than they need to be if we as teachers and TAs do not help them with visual information on timetables and in the way we visually present tasks. Other children can become prompt-dependent in that they cue into the comments of adults which occur regularly and which some children begin to expect as an integral and necessary cue or part of their routine. As teachers and TAs in a busy classroom we can sometimes be unaware of how a child on the autism spectrum is viewing our regular verbal instructions as prompts.

CASE STUDY: JAKE

Jake, a primary pupil, worked with one teaching assistant in the mornings and a different TA in the afternoon. Jake accepted this arrangement without any problem. Sometimes if the TA who worked with Jake in the mornings saw Jake in the afternoon she would say, 'Hello, Jake, how are you?' Jake would reply, 'Hello, Mrs Smith, how are you?' If Mrs Smith did not walk through the classroom Jake did not ask about her or notice but when she did they exchanged this greeting. One afternoon Mrs Smith passed quickly through the classroom and into an adjoining room from which she could be seen. As Jake was busy working she did not want to disturb him, so did not say anything. Jake became agitated when he saw her in the other room. He kept getting up and tapping on the window, calling out, 'How are you?' unable to concentrate on his work.

What might staff think the behaviour was about?
Initially staff could feel that Jake was not being co-operative or not wanting to work.

What else could it be?
Jake wanted to speak to Mrs Smith.

How did Jake's autism affect his behaviour?
Jake felt that if he saw Mrs Smith he had to speak to her and receive a reply. This was now a routine to Jake which he felt had to happen.

Children on the autism spectrum have difficulties with flexible and imaginative thinking, combined with social and communication difficulties, which results in problems understanding fact and fantasy, understanding a concept of finish, understanding what others are thinking or feeling, commonly called theory of mind.

How can we create teaching and learning opportunities from our knowledge and understanding of autism?

The general perception of the behaviours that children on the autism spectrum present within the three key areas of difficulty is that they are impairments or deficits. It is certainly true that the difficulties children on the autism spectrum display can be complex and challenging for them, making it harder for them to understand the way many other people may be following the unspoken or unwritten rules of our daily situations. However, the three areas which define autism can also be significant and helpful pointers to how those of us not on the spectrum can modify our responses so that we can be more effective in different ways of communicating which children on the autism spectrum can access. Understanding the nature of autism can help us to plan to the learning strengths of children on the spectrum, developing a range of communication, interaction and thinking patterns which help us to be clearer in what we present and expect from all pupils, not just those who have autism.

It is therefore useful to look at autism as a signpost for what we can do to be more effective practitioners. Understanding autism really helps teachers and TAs to view the behaviour of their pupils differently. Consider how the case of Stephen demonstrates this.

CASE STUDY: STEPHEN

Stephen was a child with severe ASD and severe learning difficulties. He was unable to communicate verbally. Stephen arrived in school, unpacked his bag and entered the classroom He went to his desk and picked up the first symbol on his timetable. As soon as he did this he became very angry. He hit the table and kicked his chair over.

What might staff think the behaviour was about?
Initially it might seem as if the cause of the outburst was Stephen communicating that he did not want to follow his timetable and was refusing to co-operate.

What else could it be?
A teaching assistant quickly communicated to the teacher that Stephen had not put his home–school communication book into the book box, which was part of Stephen's arrival routine.

How did Stephen's autism affect his behaviour?
Once Stephen reached the next part of his arrival routine, using his timetable to see what activity he was to do, he was unable to proceed because for him a vital step was missing and the arrival routine was not yet finished.

What could staff do to help Stephen?
As soon as Stephen was shown a home–school book he calmed. He knew that the staff understood his problem. He sat and waited, as instructed, whilst a staff member was sent to get a book which he could put in the book box. Stephen was not concerned that it was not his book, only that the routine could not be followed and completed.

This chapter asks us as teachers and TAs where we could change our perception of the 'triad of impairment' so as to see the teaching and learning opportunities that an understanding of the triad gives us as professionals in education. Each element of the triad can be more positively thought of as a difference in the way children on the spectrum interact, communicate and think flexibly. The three key areas of 'difference' help us as teachers and teaching assistants to know immediately how we can be more effective in our approach. A child on the autism spectrum learns less effectively if we maintain high levels of interaction and verbal communication. Understanding this difference immediately alerts us to recognize that a child on the autism spectrum will learn more effectively if we plan times into the school day where the child is not expected to interact and can relax, or, where he is expected to interact, ensure that he is clear what he has to do. He may be happier and more receptive to learning if he has had some times in the day when he is expected to work alone. He is a visual learner, not helped by too much language to process. Therefore to make this a teaching opportunity we need to increase our use of visual communication methods rather than the spoken word. A child on the spectrum learns less effectively if we expect him to know the usual codes of conduct and to be able to imagine what else we want him to do. He learns more effectively if we ensure that everything is clear to him about what the next step in his day, or in an activity, is. A pupil who has behaviour difficulties because we are expecting him to be more flexible than he understands how to be need not have those behaviour difficulties if we understand that we have to help him be adaptable by using visual systems in a way that ensures that changes are incorporated within them yet presented so that the child understands them, is prepared for them and is not stressed by them. If we use our understanding of autism we can plan – to have a clear finish to contexts or activities, to be clear about what is going to happen, to have times for feeling relaxed and without demands, to be warned when things are finishing or changing.

As we consider particular behaviours that an individual displays we can consider how we can use our knowledge as an opportunity. For example, if a child does not like looking at us when we are talking should we perhaps assess whether the child needs to be looking at us or whether he can listen and process more effectively without doing so.

Identifying and understanding the characteristics we see displayed within each area of difficulty is the most effective signpost we can have as educators in knowing how we can adjust and modify our interactions, our communication and our teaching methods so that they are more easily understood by children on the autism spectrum.

Mesibov *et al.* (2004) characterize the role of those working and supporting children with autism as that of a 'cross-cultural interpreter'.

TRY THIS!

Say out loud, as if to yourself, what you are doing to solve a problem rather than verbally instructing the child directly about what he should do in a situation e.g. 'This does not seem to be working. What can I do here? I think I'll try to ...', etc. Some children are more able to listen and learn indirectly than directly and may learn from teachers and TAs describing the problem-solving processes.

Teachers, teaching assistants, other professionals and parents all play vital roles in decoding hidden meanings for children on the autism spectrum.

Teachers and TAs who can decode situations and expose hidden meanings can really help such pupils.

If teachers and teaching assistants have a thorough understanding of each individual child and the way in which his behaviour and learning is being affected by each area of the triad of impairment, and also by the interrelationship of these features, they should hopefully find themselves more equipped to problem-solve and support children in what and how they learn. Interpreting autism and each child's unique profile enables us to create a triad of opportunity where we match our teaching approach to the ways in which children on the autism spectrum most effectively learn.

Suggestions for helping children with autism to learn

INTERPRETING THE AUTISM SPECTRUM AND THE TRIAD OF TEACHING OPPORTUNITY

- Develop a broad knowledge of autism.
- Develop an understanding of each individual's unique autism profile.
- Recognize the range of features and the presentation of features within each area of the triad.
- Focus on the learning strengths of a child with autism.
- Use difficulties as opportunities for understanding autism and for supporting adults in modifying interactions and communication to be effective.
- Recognize and prepare for our role as 'cross-cultural interpreter'.

FURTHER READING

- Faherty, C. (2000) *Asperger's. What does it mean to me?* Arlington TX: Future Horizons.
- Mesibov, G., Shea, V. and Schopler, E. (2004) *The TEACCH Approach to Autism Spectrum Disorders.* New York: Springer.
- Wiley, L. (1999) *Pretending to be Normal. Living with Asperger's Syndrome.* London: Jessica Kingsley.

The Autism-friendly Professional

2

This chapter focuses not on the child with autism but on the professionals who work with the child. This chapter considers:

■ What do we mean by an 'autism-friendly' professional?

■ What positive qualities and skills do parents appreciate in professionals working with a child who has autism?

■ What specific pressures do teachers and teaching assistants who work with children on the autism spectrum feel under?

■ What support do teachers and TAs find helpful when supporting children on the autism spectrum?

Children are taught by a range of people in their lives – parents or carers, other family members, teachers, teaching assistants, and by a range of other professionals. This chapter is aimed particularly at teachers and teaching assistants and those professionals involved in teaching children on the autism spectrum in the school setting. However, some of the points raised may also be relevant to those who 'teach' these children in different contexts too. Anyone involved in guiding, supporting or teaching a child on the autism spectrum can begin to see how important it is to think in an 'autism-friendly' way for children to be fully understood and taught in ways which match the way they think and learn.

What do we mean by an 'autism-friendly' professional?

To be an 'autism-friendly professional', teachers and TAs need to really understand children on the spectrum and how they can so easily misunderstand what we want from them. We also need to actively use our knowledge of autism and our understanding of each individual pupil, to be effective, both in terms of problem-solving and planning for children to learn.

'Autism-friendly professionals' find themselves needing an abundance of the very skills that children on the autism spectrum have great difficulty in acquiring or using. Teachers and teaching assistants often have to demonstrate:

- Flexibility and creativity in how they think and problem-solve.

- Empathy, insight and the ability to change their practices as they 'read between the lines' of what a child is thinking or doing.

- Good communication skills, knowing how and when to communicate.

- A high degree of organization in terms of systems and materials in order for children to learn.

- Willingness to listen, collaborate and learn from others.

Many of these skills are needed when working with other children too, but they are even more necessary when working with children on the autism spectrum, who often need powerful routines and clearly defined systems to enable them to access what is usual and obvious to most other children.

The next section of the chapter considers what the children and their parents want from the professionals who work with their child.

What positive qualities and skills do parents appreciate in professionals working with a child who has autism?

Parents of children on the autism spectrum are often looking for professionals who can really understand the unique needs of their individual child with autism. Often their first concern is whether their child is happy and calm in his classroom and school. Most parents know from experience that a child on the autism spectrum is unable to demonstrate skills and learn if he is unhappy or anxious. A child with autism who feels worried or unclear may display his stress by being unable to function at all, either becoming more and more withdrawn or displaying challenging behaviour. If a child is calm and happy this tells a parent a lot about the quality of the relationship he has with school staff and how well he is understood. Parents usually know the small details which mean a lot to their child and often feel comfortable with those professionals who want to identify what helps a child feel relaxed and able to cope.

On page 29 are a few comments from parents who were asked how their children felt about their teachers or teaching assistants. The exercise can be carried out independently, used by a class team or used as part of continuing professional development training to promote discussion.

POSITIVE PROFESSIONAL–PARENTAL PERSPECTIVES

Read the following four comments from parents. Reflect on the skills, attitude or understanding the teacher or TA has which is recognized by the parent as making a difference to their son or daughter.

Jake

loves this teacher. She understands how much his drawing means to him and how it calms him. She balances his timetable so he works hard, which he doesn't mind, but he also knows when he is allowed to draw and what time he has to do it. Just this has really helped him feel able to cope.

Alison

has a great TA. She knows that Alison is different: there is no point thinking she's not, because she is. But this TA accepts her differences in a positive way and helps the other kids to be accepting too. She knows what Alison is good at and makes sure that Alison and others are aware of it too. She makes sure that Alison does not miss out on what is going on in school either. She will prepare Alison for any things that are going to happen in school. So, by the time it happens, Alison can go along to it or join in without it distressing her.

Steven

cannot talk but there is no mistaking that he is now happy in his class. Since going into the class he is excited when he sees his school bag ready at the door. He jumps up and heads for the door the minute he sees the bus. This did not happen in his previous class. He may not be able to tell me how he feels, but his behaviour always does. I get his home–school book every night and I get told if there are any problems, but I also get told nice things and funny stories and this really helps me. I know I can write back or phone any time and speak to someone if I have any worries.

James

has two TAs now, and this has really been good for him. They both understand and like him and he knows it. The Senco is good too. The reason he feels good is that they are consistent with him and organize things the same way. If one of them is away he does not fall to bits now, as he knows that things will be ok.

Parents of children on the autism spectrum are likely to want a range of different things from the professionals who work with their child. However, from experience of working with a range of families over a number of years there have been some qualities that parents have repeatedly identified as making a professional really caring and understanding, no matter what age or school setting their child was in.

Sensitive honesty

Firstly, a number of parents commented on the need to be told information about their son or daughter honestly but to have it presented with compassion and sensitivity. One parent commented on how important it was to know what was really happening with her child.

> I always felt the teacher was telling me everything, even the worst moments my child was having in school. Although it was not great to hear, it meant I was not kept in the dark, and that I was in on the discussions about it.
>
> (Parent of a Year 4 pupil)

Parents also commented on how much easier it was to hear difficult information about their child when things were said to them in a 'caring way'.

> The way she told me things made me feel that she still liked my son. No matter what had gone on, she always made it clear that the reason for us meeting to talk about it was to try and help him. That made it much easier for me.
>
> (Parent of a child in a special school for children with severe learning difficulties)

When asked about what constituted teachers and teaching assistants talking to them in a 'caring way' parents described this as ways which did not over-dramatize the problem, suggested reasons why it might have occurred and what ideas could be tried to prevent it happening again.

Some parents felt that not being told information at the time a situation had occurred and finding out when things had become very difficult was much worse than being given the information as it happened. However, they really valued those teachers who could talk to them about a situation and present it in a way which showed how much they wanted to help the child to overcome the problem in the future.

> It never sounded from her voice or attitude that there was any criticism of my son or me. She just expressed concern about what she could do to handle things differently and help.
>
> (Parent commenting on Senco supporting Year 7 pupil)

Some parents commented on how good it was to be able to talk to the teacher about an issue rather than just read about it in a note, which sometimes led to further misunderstandings.

Respectful of parent knowledge

Teachers, TAs and parents can together make strong teams.

Some parents made comments about how much they wanted to offer suggestions and input to teachers and teaching assistants, but were not sure whether they should or not. Some parents also felt that school staff asking them for ideas made it easier for them to do the same when a problem started to arise at home.

> I really like this present teacher because although she is good and knowledgeable herself, she sometimes asks me what things I've tried. She asks me what has worked or not worked at home and I really feel like she wants my ideas.
>
> (Parent of a child in Year 1)

What specific pressures do teachers and teaching assistants feel under when working with pupils on the autism spectrum?

In order for children on the autism spectrum to learn, those who 'teach' them have to take care of themselves and be well supported by the schools in which they work. Teachers and teaching assistants who are supporting a pupil on the autism spectrum can sometimes find themselves feeling de-skilled, over-responsible, isolated or overwhelmed. It is important that schools understand how staff can feel when working with children who may require new or different levels of thinking.

What additional planning considerations or arrangements do teachers and TAs often have to consider which enable pupils on the autism spectrum to feel able to cope in school and learn?

Teachers can often feel permanently attached to a 'to do' list and there are a number of additional planning pressures when working with children with ASD. Pupils on the spectrum often require teachers and TAs to make individual arrangements for maximizing their ability to cope, understand and learn. These can include:

- Making special arrangements for routines such as break times, lunch, playtimes, etc.

- Preparing a child for educational visits or special events like Christmas, or activity weeks where the routines will be very different, etc.

- Helping the child to sit in the least distracting place in terms of social demands, or sensory difficulties such as light, sound, heat.

- Planning a timetable that includes extra one-to-one teaching times so as to familiarize the pupil with the work and reduce anxieties or with teaching concepts related to social expectations.

- Assessing, making, restructuring or maintaining the use of visual teaching tools and systems that enable the pupil to make sense of his classroom, working environments and expectations.

How can misunderstanding a child with autism affect our professional self-esteem as teachers and TAs?

Sometimes, when feeling overwhelmed, it can be difficult to talk to other colleagues about the situation or feel positive about suggestions for strategies. When feeling stressed, we can find ourselves saying and believing that a strategy 'won't work', or 'we've done that before.'

> The teacher from the Communication and Interaction team helped me. She suggested that, instead of observing just how good the child was with others, I should focus on noting down the way others spoke to him, the volume, how the instructions were given, and so on, to see what made him take notice of these people. Also she told me to write stuff down for him, instead of talking too much. These things helped me to get my own relationship with him going and my confidence came back.
>
> (Teaching assistant working with Year 8 pupil)

These feelings can be particularly strong if the pupil has regressed in behaviour and learning, as we can feel personally responsible for the child having difficulties.

Under stress, teachers and teaching assistants can find themselves feeling unable to think through the difficulties a pupil is experiencing, either behaviourally or with learning, and feel unsure where to start tackling the child's difficulties. If we are autism-friendly professionals then our attitude to behaviour difficulties can be kept in perspective if we recognize that the pupil is likely to be using his behaviour to communicate that he is unsure what is expected, or feels overwhelmed. He may be communicating that he is unfamiliar with what is happening, or feeling anxious. If we truly accept that autism is causing the child to misunderstand or misinterpret, rather than the child making any deliberate attempt to be difficult, we have an empathetic starting point for problem solving. We may be able to accept, too, that we may well be contributing to his behavioural difficulties without realizing it, or maybe unable to manage his behaviour because our usual methods are not helpful with a child who experiences life differently. Understanding how autism is affecting a child's behaviour can really de-personalize it for us and allow us to be empathetic to the child, as well as to ourselves.

> I had always been thought of by colleagues as a good teacher. I had a real belief that this child on the autism spectrum would be no different from any other child and would respond to the same methods that I had used successfully with many children with learning difficulties, even those with emotional or behavioural difficulties. I felt quite shocked and inadequate really, especially when we put our usual strategies into place and it did not get better, in fact if I'm honest it got worse.
> (Teacher in a special school for pupils with moderate learning difficulties Year 7)

If this is the case, it is important that staff are supported in making changes in their usual practices and may need specialist input where necessary to seek out the kinds of strategies which are supportive to children on the autism spectrum. Teachers and teaching assistants do not intend their expectations of a child to be part of his cumulative stress. However, they may not have had prior experience of how to balance the levels of relaxation and familiarization that a child may need to understand or cope.

Teachers and TAs may also not have used visual ways of structuring activities and routines in these ways before, and have to learn how to do so. Sometimes the cause of stress may not be directly related to the child's school experience, but may still require us to take action in school to help the student cope by temporarily lowering demands, providing more visual clarification, or adjusting his relaxation times.

TRY THIS!

Talk to the parents, and staff who have worked with the child, to find out information which helps you plan successful working times with a good balance of relaxation so that the child remains calm and not stressed. Ask questions such as:

- What does/did the child find calming to do? How frequently does/did the child need times to relax? How long does/did the child need to really relax and then be able to work again?

- Does the child work better knowing there will be a relaxation time after a work session, or does he work better when relaxation time comes first and then he is asked to work?

- How many tasks or activities can the child do comfortably? What length of time can he work for comfortably?

If the child is in a state of heightened stress, increase the number of relaxation times and the length of relaxation periods.

Some of the ways we can manage, prevent or redirect challenging behaviours to try and help the pupil are considered further in Chapter 5. In this chapter we are concerned with meeting our needs as professionals when we feel under stress in these sorts of situations.

Sometimes situations like this can make us feel unsure of our professional strengths. Stress from the additional work load of supporting a child on the autism spectrum who is displaying challenging behaviour can sometimes make us feel less understanding and less 'autism-friendly' in our approach than we would want to be. Yet it is often at these times that the pupil himself needs us to be even more understanding of his difficulties. When we are faced with temper outbursts and upsets from pupils on the autism spectrum it is difficult for us to remain calm and be focused on what we can do. We can sometimes feel that other colleagues are considering us weak or unable to maintain discipline. We can begin to see the difficulty in terms of discipline and behaviour management, rather than in terms of a child with autism who may be confused, upset, angry or without the necessary knowledge or skills to do things differently. By considering the behaviour from the perspective of autism we can see how difficult it is for the pupil as well as his school staff or family.

What support do teachers and TAs find helpful when supporting children on the autism spectrum?

Effective teamwork

Children on the autism spectrum benefit from a whole range of professionals supporting their education and working with their families to maximize their learning. Teachers, TAs,

Sencos, other professionals, parents and the pupils themselves can all be useful contributors to our wider teams. Good teams can provide really positive support to each other and to the pupil.

> When Josh first moved to our school he was having a really difficult time, and we were trying to find out what worked with him. So while we tried things we looked out for each other. We shared roles in supporting him. Sometimes if we could see things were getting difficult we would change over staff to help each other out and make sure we had the energy and the patience to calmly support him.
>
> (Senco: Year 3 pupil)

Keeping each member of our team contributing can ensure we share the work load. It is important to share knowledge within a team about areas of expertise associated with our roles. Often parents have knowledge and information to share about what has been successful or not successful in the past.

Teaching assistants can sometimes focus on observing detailed information which may help identify specifically what a child finds difficult or helpful.

> He used to call out or try and talk to me when lessons were being introduced and did not seem to understand that he should be listening to the teacher in that bit. He likes to doodle, and I realized that if I let him do this during the time the teacher was talking it helped him sit quietly and, more importantly, listen. When the teacher asked questions at the end, he was able to answer them. Now whoever works with him encourages this, and it's seen as a helpful strategy, not a cop-out.
>
> (Teaching assistant: Year 5)

Some pupils are also capable of providing information about themselves. Written sheets of suggested reasons or options that a student can select from to give their understanding of their own needs can often give us vital insights.

For example, with more able pupils on the autism spectrum a written or symbol-supported worksheet asking a child what he especially likes doing can be used every half-term to ensure that we remain in touch with any changes in a pupil's special interests.

Sometimes when pupils are experiencing periods of real anxiety or distress because of major life changes or events over which they or we have little control it is important to ensure that they have a routine and some work structures that they are able to easily achieve success with but which are not too demanding. Establishing a classroom coping routine which has higher structure than usually required and lower demands in terms of academic challenges can be useful as a short-term survival position should a pupil require it.

What can help teachers and TAs to establish efficient team work?

There is often so much to be done in school and in a short time span. When supporting children on the autism spectrum the more prepared staff are in their use of visual information and instructions the more independence the pupil will have in the classroom. Teachers and TAs therefore need to put more time into preparation so that they need to do less explaining while working because the way they have set up an activity gives the pupil the level of communication about what to do already.

To be good at planning for greater independence in learning, and preparing materials which tell the pupil what to do by the way they are set up and presented, teachers and TAs need to be good at managing their preparation time.

Sometimes we need simple meeting formats that can help us be time-efficient yet focused on improving the behaviour and learning opportunities of the child. When we are short on time we sometimes forget to consider what is going well with a pupil, yet it is important to spend a few moments establishing this, both for the morale of the staff and also because it can provide clues as to what factors are particularly helpful for an individual child.

- What is going well and why?

- What is difficult at present and why?

- What changes could we make or strategies could we try to help the child create a new response? (List them all as ideas.)

- Which strategy matches what we already know or where do we need to know more information?

Where behaviour and learning are going well with a child we may need to focus on a different set of meeting questions such as:

- How can we extend this pupil's level of independence?

- Where can we generalize or teach flexibility?

Sometimes pupils on the autism spectrum need teaching aspects which we might refer to as the hidden curriculum. They may need to be taught social skills or to be provided with to be taught information about situations that other pupils would not require help to understand. Sometimes these elements are vital 'life skills' for pupils on the autism spectrum. Teachers, TAs, parents and other professionals who work together as a team can give each other support in selecting and prioritizing what is really helpful for a child on the autism spectrum to learn. Teams who understand that a child on the autism spectrum requires an educational programme which balances aspects of teaching the hidden curriculum as well as the main curriculum can be very supportive to each other. Teams who understand the impact of autism on a pupil can focus their teaching and educational goals on what would really help the child even when this may not be convenient to the usual arrangements, or easily understood by other colleagues.

Sometimes teachers and teaching assistants really need to meet and discuss points of action, and other times points can be communicated perhaps in other ways. Page 38 shows a simple format which can be used to record the action to be taken following a meeting or may replace a meeting in some situations where the action to be taken is about assessing and finding out information from which to create a strategy. (This example is followed by a blank form which readers can photocopy and use themselves.)

The key points to consider in planning an intervention are *what* needs doing, *why* it needs doing to ensure everyone understands the purpose of the action, *who* will be responsible for carrying out which parts of it and *when* it will be carried out.

Professionals who work well together can help each other to predict times when a pupil may have particular problems and can try to plan for them so that major difficulties can be avoided. For example, is important for teachers and TAs to allow a pupil time to familiarize himself with school and classroom structures and systems for the first week or two after a school holiday break. Sometimes if teachers or TAs do not allow a short period of readjustment into school routines and educational demands a pupil can begin to feel anxious and begin displaying behaviour difficulties, which might be avoided by careful planning and reintroduction to the use of visual supports and systems.

Sometimes more able pupils may say, 'This is easy. I know this,' when demands are at a level which the child is coping well with. Rather than feel that we have failed to offer a challenging level of work for the child, it can be a sign that the pupil is comfortable and not stressed. With careful step by step planning we will make progress more quickly, by familiarizing the pupil in this way.

Whole-school support and planning: establishing consistent approaches built on a sound knowledge of autism

Wider aspects of school life can be crucial in supporting pupils who are on the autism spectrum. For school life to be meaningful in and beyond the classroom for pupils with autism it is important for schools to produce clear policies and structures. Schools can demonstrate proactive approaches to supporting both pupils and their staff, so that special arrangements are in place for aspects of school life such as transition from school to school or special arrangements for lunch or break times. Whole-school strategies can also be essential for providing a positive ethos, from which parents and professionals can collaborate to support pupils.

Schools which have clear 'autism-friendly' policy statements addressing issues such as effective teaching approaches, or how autism can affect behaviour, provide their school staff with supportive guidelines which enable them to function within a whole-school approach.

Consulting staff across the school, when creating proactive policies, ensures that teachers and TAs have ownership and that policies have consistency. The exercise on page 40 suggests statements about the use of visual strategies such as written or picture information to help children on the autism spectrum learn.

TEACHER/TEACHING ASSISTANT: ACTION PLAN

What	Why	Who	When
Establish an independent work file for Tony. 1 Gather worksheets and activities the student likes to do and can already do. 2 Prepare file folder with a work to do section and a finished work section.	To teach independent work/study skills. To prevent the pupil becoming overwhelmed and exhibiting behaviour difficulties in some lessons.	TA to collect worksheets and activities. Student could help with photocopying the materials and sorting into subjects for ease of storage and reference. Teacher and Senco to set up how it will be used.	Week beginning 6 January. Use one-to-one work time before lunch on Tuesday and Thursday. Use Friday p.m. assembly time to review it ready for use the following week.
Establish a strategy for dealing with Jason's difficult behaviour after lunch. 1 Try giving Jason some down time on entry to the classroom with his reading book for five minutes. 2 Let Jason review the afternoon timetable before he starts lessons. Put in a short mid-afternoon quiet time.	To try and prevent or reduce afternoon outbursts and enable Jason to focus in afternoon lessons. See if this calms him and gives him time to prepare for the afternoon. We do this in the morning and perhaps he needs this overview in the p.m. too?	TA to consult with teacher on playground duty each day to find out any information about incidents during lunch. Teacher and TA to review if this strategy reduces or eliminates afternoon outbursts.	Week beginning: Review end of following week.

TEACHER/TEACHING ASSISTANT : ACTION PLAN

What	Why	Who	When

VISUAL TOOLS: FROM POLICY TO PRACTICE

The statements below could be enlarged, photocopied and cut into separate statements. Staff can be asked to rewrite them to reflect their beliefs.

The rewritten statements can be shared and then given to the teacher responsible for writing a policy statement.

This approach could be used to help school staff create policy statements relating to other aspects of teaching and learning for children with autism too.

Rewrite the following statements so they reflect your practice:

■ Every student with autism should be using a visual tool.

■ Only pictures are useful to convey information.

■ Visual strategies are to be used only in the classroom.

■ Good teaching relies upon the use of visual approaches.

■ Symbols should be standardized and the same ones used for each pupil and through-out the school.

■ Visual symbols should be obvious without being explained or pupils having to be taught their use.

■ Visual symbols are OK for younger pupils but older pupils do not need them.

As children on the autism spectrum are visual learners, many teachers and teaching assistants understand that using visual approaches can be a major part of a positive teaching and learning ethos. 'Visual approaches' are ways that can be used to tackle a problem, ensuring that a child 'sees' what he needs to do or understands rather than relying on verbal explanations. We all use techniques for remembering events, organizing our daily or weekly timetables in the form of written lists, diaries, calendars, etc. Visual approaches are particularly supportive in providing for children and older students who find it difficult to listen, concentrate, remember, process language or organize their own needs. Many children on the autism spectrum have combinations of these difficulties and particularly tend to find language more confusing than clarifying when trying to understand what others are saying or want of them. Receiving messages and thinking in picture images is quite often a preferred mode of operation for people on the autism spectrum and a strength area.

Over time it may become clear which kinds of visual tools work effectively with a child. This can become a regular visual strategy and part of an essential lifelong approach to teaching social and coping skills.

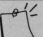

TRY THIS!

Before spending a lot of time making a resource, test out whether it will be helpful to a child first.

Make a 'rough' version of the resource, e.g. an initial handwritten instruction rather than a typed one.

Next try it out, assess whether it will help the child.

Then work on:

- What might individualize it to make it more effective?
- What will enable it to have flexibility?
- What will make it longer-lasting, substantial and well presented?

It is important to consider that the word 'visual' should mean that anyone looking at what we present can understand the message quickly and easily, without any language being used verbally to explain it. Sometimes when we use visual tools we can minimize their initial impact by putting verbal instructions or explanations with them immediately. Although teachers and teaching assistants often know that children on the autism spectrum are visual learners and tend to respond better to visual than verbal direction they still tend to use language as their first medium of communication and if this fails they continue to use it rather than reducing or not using spoken language. Using written words, pictures or objects to convey to students essential meaning should, as 'autism-friendly' professionals, be our priority in communicating to and with our pupils.

Suggestions for helping children with autism to learn

BEING AN 'AUTISM-FRIENDLY' PROFESSIONAL

- Explore and inform your own beliefs about how children usually learn and where children on the autism spectrum learn differently.

- Work with the pupil, parents and other professionals to predict potential times which may require careful planning.

- Be able to step back, de-personalize and reflect on your own actions and how a child on the spectrum may read or misread them.

- Create and use staff support systems and school or class policies.

FURTHER READING

- Plimley, L. and Bowen M. (2006) *Supporting Pupils with Autistic Spectrum Disorders. A Guide for School Support Staff.* London: Paul Chapman Publishing.

- Plimley, L. and Bowen, M. (2007) *Social Skills and Autistic Spectrum Disorders.* London: Paul Chapman Publishing.

Making Sense of Changes and Transitions

This chapter considers in depth one particular area of difficulty for children on the autism spectrum, understanding and accepting changes in daily routines and situations. The chapter looks at:

- What we mean by 'change'.

- A range of autism perspectives on 'change'.

- The relationship between 'change and stress'.

- Transitions as a key component of 'change'.

- Ways of teaching children to understand and accept change.

What is this chapter about?

Everyone experiences changes occurring in their daily lives on a large or small scale. Consequently we all recognize that 'changes" can happen in a number of forms and demand different responses from us. Changes in our lives can be the result of major life events or may be the accumulation of small readjustments day to day.

Changes can be positive in that we want them to happen or are glad they happened, just as they can be challenging or unexpected. The intensity, frequency, pace and duration of changes which occur for each of us at different times in our lives vary, as does the way each person copes with, enjoys or tolerates changes, and whether we view changes as positive or negative.

Problems with flexible and imaginative thinking are a key area of difficulty for children on the autism spectrum. This chapter explores the complexities of understanding and accepting changes which we can all experience, but which children on the autism spectrum find particularly difficult. By providing time for children to get used to different places, activities and ways of doing things they can be better prepared to understand, predict and respond to changes. The chapter also focuses on how teachers, TAs and other adults involved in supporting children with autism have to use clear structures and systems to help children learn but also have a responsibility to use those systems flexibly with the child, so that rigidity is gently challenged and not reinforced by us.

What do we mean by change?

Change literally means something is different from how it was. Some of, or all, the elements of a situation have been altered, replaced, removed, converted, transformed or substituted so that it is no longer the same.

When we find ourselves in different or unexpected situations or circumstances that require us to respond in a way we have not done before, and which we have no routine response to, we can have some small insight and empathy with the feelings that children or adults on the autism spectrum may encounter when they experience changes in what they were expecting to happen. When thinking about how we respond to changes or new experiences we can find ourselves saying things like 'I feel out of my comfort zone,' or ' I've done things this way for so long that I feel unsure of myself doing them differently.'

If the changes taking place are very major then we may require some time to think things through, and consider how we feel about the changes, and to adjust. We can find that when changes occur quickly, one after another, or the change is very intense and demanding on our coping reserves, their effect upon us can be quite stressful.

If the changes are expected to some degree, we often seem to be able to plan ahead and respond in an appropriate way, rearrange and be flexible to accommodate differences. If the changes are minor but cumulative in nature, then sometimes we can also experience some difficulty in responding to them and the level of stress can gradually build.

We may find that the changes that occur in our daily lives or in life events can sometimes be a positive experience and help us to break free of old habits and responses which we may have felt consciously or subconsciously are controlling us more than we wanted them to.

One of the factors that makes 'change' situations positive for us is when we clearly understand the reasons for the changes and can exert some degree of control over them rather than changes being imposed upon us. These insights into our own responses provide us with some empathy for the very real difficulties that children on the autism spectrum experience.

What makes changes occurring particularly difficult for people on the autism spectrum?

Some children on the autism spectrum find it difficult to perceive what is expected of them in new situations and this difficulty in predicting what will be asked of them can contribute to a child's anxieties about change. A child with autism may not be able to 'imagine' what else he could do when he finds himself suddenly in circumstances of which he has no visual memory and consequently no routine response for. Other children seem to be unaware and unable to anticipate, while others appear to be over-anxious about anticipating what is next if given the information too far in advance.

Some children on the autism spectrum actively resist changes which they do not understand, and this often results in distressed or challenging behaviour. It can be helpful for teachers, TAs and other professionals, parents or carers to have a knowledge of the range of ways that children on the autism spectrum may perceive change. From this knowledge it is useful to observe and identify each child's individual response to changes, so that the knowledge can be used to support each child in the way we present change and teach the child to be flexible.

Sometimes it is clear to us that the child is finding a particular situation difficult, because there are obvious factors involved, and ones that teachers, TAs or others can see might be problematic and require the child to get used to e.g. a different teacher or TA, different room, different group, etc. Other times it is difficult to recognize what exactly the child is seeing as changed, but for a child with severe autism any small detail may have been omitted which makes the situation unrecognizable or only partly as they expected it to be.

In some situations there are partial changes in that some factors are still the same and others are different. There are some children on the autism spectrum who find partial changes more difficult than completely new situations. Completely new situations or routines which are not recognized can sometimes fill a child with anxieties because he does not know what to do. For other children on the spectrum they provide an opportunity to start again. With no strong visual memories to draw on, the child accepts new situations and learns what he has to do. It is only later when he visually recalls the pattern of what he has to do that he notices changes.

Among children who do respond better to 'new' situations, gradual or partial changes can make some feel very insecure because they may recognize people, places or features from an old situation. In the new one they are unsure whether they should be following old routines or whether they are to follow a new routine.

Other children do not display behaviour challenges but experience stress inwardly and may become withdrawn when feeling unsure of changes. Some children faced with transitions may be passive resisters in that they comply slowly and may create a routine for the transition which is subtle and appropriate. Sharon was a quiet girl who never got angry and always tried to do the right thing when asked. Whenever activities finished and the class were asked to assemble in the corner area or get ready for the next activity, she was always last to arrive in the place where the activity was to take place, and as she packed things away she would straighten all the pencils in the pencil pots as part of her own transition routine.

Digging deeper into what signifies a 'change' to an individual child on the autism spectrum

It can be difficult to understand why sometimes a child finds a change easier to accept than we would anticipate and at other times a change in the routine causes major distress. Sometimes a child may not react with upset because he finds himself in an entirely new routine or a new set of circumstances. He therefore has no visual memory of the new situations and is not anticipating what should happen or trying to recreate sameness.

For something to be a change it has to be recognized or remembered in its former state. If a situation is totally different it is not actually a change but something new, and this can be the reason why some situations may be accepted by children with ASD. The situations are not ones they have visual memories of.

> Kyle does not like minor changes in class routines and so we were concerned about him moving to a class where there would be significant differences in what he would be expected to do. In the first few weeks he has surprised us, as he's been very calm and no problem at all. We're wondering if this just suits him better, or maybe it's a lull before the storm.
>
> (Teacher and TA working with Year 2 pupil)

Equally, when trying to change how a child behaves it can be important to start a new routine very definitely before a child with autism enters an existing behaviour routine. Once the child begins a known routine he may become compulsive in carrying it out. Therefore any changes we are trying to make will not be accepted easily.

CASE STUDY: PETER

Peter, a boy with autism and moderate learning difficulties in Year 3, was upset when a child from another class, Tony, tried to take his picture cards to look at during lunchtime. At the end of the day all classes assembled to leave on school transport. When Peter saw the other child looking at him at the assembly point, he hit him. The next day at the transport assembly point Peter repeated this behaviour. Within a few days it was Peter's regular response. He also became angry with staff if they tried to stop him or told him not to.

What might staff think the behaviour was about?
This behaviour appeared on the surface to be quite vengeful and aggressive, with Peter continuing a vendetta against Tony.

What else could it be?
The teachers and TAs who knew Peter well began to think that when Peter had seen Tony looking at him he was unsure if Tony was going to take his cards again. Also his visual memory of the incident was triggered. They decided initially, to move Tony so he was waiting in a different place, and they changed where Peter sat and waited, as they hoped it would mean Peter did not see the other child straight away. This was a good idea, and might well have worked, except that Peter had quickly established a routine of events leading up to trying to hit Tony, and it was difficult to stop him feeling compelled to do it. When Tony was moved, Peter reacted by running around looking for him, hitting out at staff and other children as he did so.

continued

How did Peter's autism affect his behaviour?

The staff had tried to make a change to redirect this behaviour. Had the behaviour been less established this could have helped. After further discussion staff realized that his behaviour had become compulsive and Peter was unable to stop. From Peter's perspective as a child with autism, he now had a hometime routine which included hitting another child. After one occasion he had established a strong and compulsive chain of events, and now felt he 'must' hit this particular child as part of his hometime routine. Intervening once Peter had started on this routine resulted only in more upset and anger. To solve the difficulty a change had to be made to the circumstances *before* Peter started the chain of events.

What did staff do to help Peter?

Staff tracked back through their usual packing-away and getting-ready-for-home routine. As they considered this they noticed that Peter began getting edgy and quick-moving around the time they packed away. They concluded that he was already in a high anxiety state and getting ready for his home routine. To prevent this they made some changes to their last lessons, the order of events for hometime and the route they took to the assembly point. The staff effectively created a new routine which Peter did not recognize and did not associate with the old one. He found this 'change' a positive experience in that the new routine enabled him to behave differently. The staff were amazed when, the first time they did this, Peter was calm and behaved well. The situation helped staff to understand what to do with Peter on future occasions where he was unable to stop or change his behaviour.

There is a whole range of factors that can indicate changes in the school context, from a new person in the classroom to changes in the school environment or changes in routines.

There is a need to consider how individual pupils may perceive change and to help professionals develop creative strategies and resources to teach effective coping skills which may have a positive effect on their behaviour, and their ability to access the curriculum.

Transitions as a key component of 'change'

For children on the autism spectrum, transitions are a key component of change. Transitions are the period of time when things change from one stage or state to another.

Transitions signify the ending of one situation, activity, setting, etc., and the start of another.

As transition times are often less defined as to what happens it can be hard for a child with autism to be focused and know what he needs to pay attention to and do. Transitions in the school environment can include a number of different parts of the day, such as coming into or going out of the classroom, moving from class to group or individual work situations, packing away materials, etc.

The relationship between transitions, change and stress

Events which require us to reassess and readjust can cause stress. Individual differences in personality and coping reserves, along with a knowledge and experience of using coping strategies to manage stress, may all be causes of distress for all of us.

Stress can be a useful feedback message and a positive energy resource. Without the right individual level of relaxation to accompany it, it becomes a negative experience. Prolonged periods of stress without time to recuperate can cause cumulative distress.

The physical effect of stress on our bodies means that we prepare ourselves for 'fight or flight' response. Our hormones activate and elevate in order to provide us with the chemical energy to cope with possible or actual threats or difficulties. The physical symptoms of stress are often a raised temperature, sometimes sweating, an increased heart rate and blood pressure, sometimes not feeling well, listlessness and a feeling of tiredness and not wanting to be bothered, a headache or nausea can also be physical signs. If we are unable physically to respond and burn off our 'fight or flight' hormones the result is a build-up of stress. If adaptive energy reserves are continually used up it is difficult to maintain our resistance to illness and our coping strategies for even more minor stresses.

Subtle changes in our daily routines may have little impact on those of us not on the autism spectrum while for someone on the autism spectrum, they may become very significant and feel much more unpredictable. The amount of questions, decisions and situations which demand new responses from people on the autism spectrum can lead to accumulative stress.

Children on the autism spectrum are likely to experience a high degree of stress due to the interrelationship of their difficulties and due to the anxieties they encounter with understanding and accepting changes. If a child with autism has become unco-operative in most, if not all, situations it means that the level of stress has overwhelmed him and become an underlying cause of challenging behaviour. Sometimes children with autism become so stressed that even visual tools, such as timetables, which usually lend support, begin to appear like demands to the child. Chapter 5 considers challenging behaviour in more detail but it is worth mentioning it here in relation to children misunderstanding changes or being unable to predict or imagine what they need to do in a given situation.

What approaches can be used to teach children to make sense of transitions and changes?

There are a number of approaches that teachers and TAs can use in the school context to help children feel more settled about transitions and changes. In this section we will be considering how to provide meaningful strategies that help children cope.

Some useful support can be provided by using the following strategies:

- Routines.

- Familiarization.

- Visual warnings.

- Factual information.

- Guided choice.

Routines

Routines can be a powerful way for children on the autism spectrum to feel sure of what they are expected to do. Routines by definition have features which children on the autism spectrum feel comfortable with, and they are an important way for teachers and TAs to provide concrete arrangements for periods of transition.

Routines generally do not vary. They are the usual way to do something, a procedure that is regularly used to perform a specific function. When a child on the autism spectrum embarks on a familiar routine he can continue anticipating what he needs to do by using his strong visual memory.

Where routines are not well defined by teachers or teaching assistants and are rarely the same, a child is likely to be confused and have no concrete clues to help him function. Some children on the autism spectrum create their own routines in situations where they do not know what to do, and this can become difficult. One of the important balances that professionals and parents have to get right for children on the autism spectrum is the balance of what needs to remain clear and constant with ensuring that we teach children to have structures that enable flexibility as well.

Routines for younger children, those in self-contained special classes, or those in a primary settings, could include arrival, going home, packing away materials, going out to the playground or to lunch, moving in and out of learning settings such as one-to-one teaching, small-group work, whole-class learning, etc. For older pupils in the secondary setting routines could include registration, homework hand-in, moving from classroom to classroom, using the canteen, etc.

Routines are repetitive, regular practices which link the day together and often provide clear markers for pupils with autism about their day. Routines provide the pupil with structures or systems to move from one activity to another or one lesson to another and provide structures which support transitions.

Children on the autism spectrum often feel more comfortable in schools where routines are clearly defined. Such routines often enable children with autism to cope with the actual lesson time because the routines are familiar to them and often provide clear start and finish signals.

Routines are useful for children with autism, where we have set them up and we are actively using them to enable a child to make transitions and to have clear expectations. However, routines are sometimes created by children with autism themselves to help them cope in particular situations, and these can cause difficulties. If we make a new routine start before a child recognizes or enters an established one we can sometimes prevent a behaviour difficulty from occurring.

Familiarization

When we feel anxious about a new situation we tend to need to familiarize ourselves with it. It is no different for children, young people and adults who are on the autism spectrum. Familiarization means spending time getting used to something. Teachers and TAs can plan to familiarize children to slowly accept new circumstances, strategies or activities.

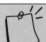

TRY THIS!

When introducing 'new' work, or 'new' subject topics, to a child on the autism spectrum try providing a short 'take a look' time for the child to look through a new book or activity, before asking questions about it.

Suggesting that teachers and TAs should familiarize a child with settings or materials and gradually build a pupil's confidence in this way sounds somewhat vague and not that important a strategy. In fact recognizing that a child may need familiarization enables teachers and TAs to plan the process and consequently set out to plan in teaching time directly for familiarization. This in turns slows down the pace at which we expect children to learn and ensures that we spend time during the familiarization period observing and assessing how a child is responding and making adjustments so that the pupil gains confidence and wants to be independent in a particular situation or with certain materials. When a child on the autism spectrum understands or has grown familiar with expectations he will often demonstrate this by being more independent and able to show his knowledge or skills.

Giving pupils who are on the autism spectrum time to get used to what is expected of them in a situation can be a very important part of successful introduction to new activities:

■ Getting used to new settings.

■ Getting used to new activities and materials.

■ Getting used to components of a strategy.

Getting used to new settings

If a child is to get to a new classroom, school, educational visit, or other venue, it could be beneficial to familiarize him with these settings. Depending on their level of understanding, children can be familiarized with new settings in a number of ways. Some children require opportunities to physically visit new settings, initially going when there are few people or activities, then further visits as necessary. For some children using photographs of them in the new setting can help. For other children using pictures, web sites, written and picture information about new settings and who the child may meet there can all help establish familiarity.

TRY THIS!

When a child will be working with new staff, not prevuiously known to him, help the child to get used to who these people are.

- If the child can read, ask new staff to wear name badges at first.
- If the child can recognize photos, use them to familiarize him with new people.
- Other ways of ensuring that he feels confortable with new people is to give new members of staff key information about the child's interests so that something relating to them can be incorporated into the initial work sessions, so as to put the child at ease, e.g. some pictures of his favourite character.

The following case studies provide examples of where teachers, teaching assistants and carers have found inventive ways to help children get accustomed to new settings and situations. The examples are not intended to provide exact solutions, only to show how the principle of familiarization can be carried out in a number of ways with a variety of individual children on the autism spectrum.

CASE STUDY : ADAM

Adam, a child in Year 1, found it hard to sit with his peers for any class lessons in the corner mat area. He would often pinch his TA and try to run off to the other side of the room.

What might staff think the behaviour was about?
Staff could view this behaviour as unwillingness to sit and work with his peers.

What else could it be?
Adam could be stressed about sitting in the mat area because he had no way of knowing how long he would be there and he may have found sitting in the midst of his peers difficult to tolerate.

How did autism affect his behaviour?
As a child with autism, Adam might find it hard to sit in close proximity to others, especially when unclear about what he was there for.

What did staff do to help?
Adam was allowed to sit on his own carpet tile a little away from the others but still in the general mat area. His TA also made him a card which showed him what was going to happen during the carpet time lesson. This involved simple card with three or four pictures indicating a combination of activities such as story, songs, numbers or letter games, etc. This way Adam could remove a card each time that section of the lesson was finished and could see progress through it, along with a picture of what happened after it, e.g. playtime or snack, etc.

If the child is staying in a new place, as some do on residential school trips, or other children in special class settings might stay at a family respite centre, then again it is important to establish familiarity with the setting as described on the previous page.

CASE STUDY : DEVON

Devon, a pupil in Year 6, along with other pupils in his class received information about the school residential planned for the summer term. He made comments about the trip to his family, his teacher and TA, saying things like, 'The school trip is going to be good, isn't it?' or 'Am I going to sleep in a new place?' As each day passed Devon repeated these things more and more and became hard to distract from the subject.

What might staff think the behaviour was about?
Initially staff were pleased that Devon seemed excited about the school trip.

What else could it be?
As time passed staff began to realize that his comments were distracting him from concentrating on his school work. It began to occur to them that Devon was anxious about the school trip and was seeking reassurance rather than expressing his excitement.

How did autism affect his behaviour?
When listening to the comments that Devon made it became more and more obvious that he was repeating what other people had said to him about the trip and was not really conveying his own thoughts. He was using their comments because as a child on the autism spectrum he did not have the communication skills to ask questions and express his anxieties about it. His difficulties as a child with autism also meant that he could not 'imagine' what it would be like on the trip unless he was familiarized with it in a more concrete way.

What did staff do to help?
Devon worked with his TA to produce a book about where the class would be staying and what they would be doing on their school residential trip. This book was shown to all the class and used by everyone to look at pictures of where they were going, how they travelled there, what children could bring with them, where they would sleep and what activities they would do each day. All the pupils in the class found the book useful, and this made Devon very involved in what the whole class was doing. He also made an individual book which contained information about things he liked to do at home to relax and had information from his parents about routines that helped him, such as his night-time routine. This level of preparation enabled Devon to be ready for and enjoy this experience.

As well as going to new contexts on school residential trips some children on the autism spectrum, particularly those in special schools, go to stay at respite centres on a regular basis. It is important for children who attend respite to maintain three-way communication between home, school and the respite centre, so as to share helpful and positive routines and other supportive strategies and resources that can help them to feel relaxed in all the settings.

CASE STUDY : JOEY

Joey, a nine-year-old boy in a special school, began attending a respite centre once a week. As he had to share a place with other children also needing such provision the plan was that he would go home after the evening meal one week and the next week would sleep the night at the respite centre. Joey behaved well on his first night but on the second occasion when he was to sleep there he was very restless and staff had a hard time getting him to go to bed.

What might staff think the behaviour was about?
Staff could have felt that Joey was testing them out and finding his boundaries.

What else could it be?
It was also important to consider that Joey did not understand he was staying the night, as on the first occasion he had gone home after teatime.

How did autism affect his behaviour?
Joey was following the routine of his first visit and had no meaningful clues that next time involved sleeping at the respite house.

What did staff do to help?
The staff carefully considered how to ensure that both these nights had very distinct and concrete clues so that Joey understood from the outset whether he was staying or not. In talking to Joey's parents it seemed that he had special slippers with his favourite cartoon character on, which he usually wore at home. If Joey was to stay the night at the respite he was taught to take his overnight bag to his bedroom, change into his slippers and put his pyjamas out on the bed. This gave him meaningful cues that he was to sleep there. If Joey was going home that night after tea he brought a different bag and was instructed to put it next to the door of the respite centre on a hook with a picture of his family on it. When he did not enter the bedroom or put on his slippers Joey became clear that it was not a night when he was going to stay there.

Getting used to activities and materials

Pupils with ASD benefit from being given some time to familiarize themselves with materials before being expected to show what they can do with them.

> The Senco suggested that I always use one-to-one teaching times to assess and teach new skills or unseen work and then move these into the classroom once practised. This has made a real difference to his confidence and we have noticed that he has fewer upsets in the class since we have been teaching in one-to-one sessions and generalizing or extending those same skills in the classroom.
>
> (Teacher and TA working with Year 6 pupil)

Sometimes TAs work with a child on the autism spectrum for one-to-one teaching sessions which focus on following up retrospectively what was being taught in lessons.

TRY THIS!

Instead of using one-to-one teaching sessions to follow up on lesson content, try using the one-to-one teaching times to focus on future lesson content. This allows a child time to familiarize himself with what he is going to be learning and may enable him to participate more fully in whole-class lessons.

When teaching children with autism and severe learning difficulties in self-contained classrooms or special schools the introduction of new activities or lesson content can be a difficult yet vital balance to get right. It can be helpful if the lesson is initially brief, with the focus on showing materials and activities rather than expecting participation or knowledge, unless a pupil shows that he is ready. Once children with severe autism and learning difficulties become less anxious about what is being asked of them they can often respond and show their skills, This teaching technique is not a lowering of expectations but a way of enabling pupils to access the skills and knowledge they already have.

Warning signals

Just as children on the autism spectrum need to be fully engaged to concentrate their attention, they also often need time to disengage where they are engrossed in an activity.

Sometimes children require a warning that there is to be an end to an activity or that they need to move on. Some children can prepare themselves for situations changing with a verbal warning: 'Caitlin, in five minutes we will be ...' For other pupils any verbal warning may disrupt their thinking or they find processing the information difficult. Visual warnings which do not require verbal explanations can be useful for some children. In considering the use of visual warnings teachers and TAs have to assess for each individual pupil how much warning is useful in preparing for change and to ensure that any strategy used helps reduce anxiety rather than increase it.

Figure 2 overleaf shows examples of the sort of visual warning cards that can be used with children who are readers. Of course the top one should be red, the middle one yellow or orange and the lowest one green. They can be photocopied on coloured card, and can be laminated so they can be written on or drawn on to clarify time limits, etc. They need to be a visual communication in that they are presented without an accompanying verbal instruction to just allow the child to recognize the 'traffic lights' colour code or read the message and prepare to finish an activity. The cards can be used consecutively in that 'Go' can let the child know on his timetable that he will be having some time that he finds fun or is free of demands. The 'Finishing soon' card can be a warning that allows time to accept that the activity is coming to an end before the 'Stop' card ends the activity. The length of time between giving out the cards is an important part of the individualizing of this strategy. The child needs to be taught to go to where his timetable is and exchange his red 'Stop' card for a green 'Go' which the teacher or teaching assistant can put back on the timetable so that he knows when the event will next occur.

Other materials for visually warning children how long they have in a situation or with a favourite activity can be sand timers or time timers, both of which are visual and have no sound. For other children a kitchen timer clock with a bell, or a digital watch with a sound signal, is more effective.

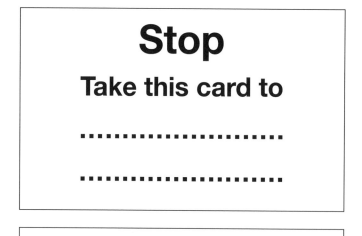

Figure 2 The sort of visual warning cards that can be used with children who can read

Relaxation

Teaching children how to relax and providing times for relaxation can be important in helping them to reduce stress and be ready for learning. One way of teaching relaxation can be to help a child learn how to breathe in and out slowly. Some pupils also benefit from going to a quiet area and doing a low-key activity which they enjoy, such as looking at a book.

In school settings, relaxation or calm areas can be established, whereas at home this might be the young person's bedroom. When out visiting friends or family it might be a designated chair, room or area that he is told about as the place he can go to when he needs some quiet time.

Security objects or special interests often provide children with consistency in a world where people, places and expectations are always in a state of change.

Time with special interests

Special interests are activities, topics or actions that a child on the autism spectrum especially enjoys doing, would rather do or talk about than anything else, and which the child usually feels comfortable with and absorbed by, and so able to engage with them and not be concerned about other events. If a child is engaged fully with his special interest, he may therefore also find it difficult to disengage when it is time to move on.

The child in this situation could feel anxious because he does not know the answer to one or more of the following questions:

- *Will I have this activity again? If so, when?* A timetable can help to indicate when the child will spend time on the activity again, which may make the transition easier for him.

- *I have not finished it to the point I wanted to. How long have I got left?* A verbal or visual warning or countdown can help if this is the difficulty.

- *What am I leaving this to go and do?* A timetable again can help a child to understand what comes next.

When making use of special interests it can be worth considering how some special-interest activities need more time than others. A child can become so engrossed that not to let them have time to engage fully and then to ask them to disengage quickly can cause more stress rather than help decrease it. In these situations it can be better to save longer spells when the child can do the activity without interruption while assessing other activities that he quite enjoys. Time can be saved by the pupil, too, towards a favourite activity which can be placed in the school week or day at convenient places where they can enjoy it more fully. If the child enjoys time on the computer, then saving picture tokens of the computer on a card towards time on it can still make it visual and motivating. An alternative can be to do an activity associated with the main interest. For example, if a student really wants to go on the computer and search for types of washing machines, but it is not possible, then a booklet of washing machine pictures from catalogues and magazines can be made up that the child can use at points during the day.

Special interests need to be reviewed regularly to ensure that they are still powerful motivators. If the child is more able, then ask him to write down his current interests; if he is not able to do this, observe his engagement with his interest, as it is important information which helps us to motivate the child or even find a way of teaching new concepts. Often when familiarizing a child with a new concept using his special interest can mean he attends carefully and becomes accustomed to the concept before working on it in other ways.

Factual information

Facts are non-emotional, clear and defined. Consequently for more able pupils with autism they are a source of valuable information from which they can prepare themselves for changes in usual events. For most pupils who can read with understanding, writing down the facts of a situation can really help.

After many difficulties John, a Year 9 student, had settled into a productive period of work, following a full timetable shared between two teaching assistants. John got on with both the teaching assistants and seemed to have settled well. Within a month of each other both TAs were planning to leave the school for different reasons. Everyone was concerned as to how John would accept these changes. Writing the facts of the situation was an effective way of planning for the change of staff. John was told when each person was leaving, what they were going to do when they left and who was replacing them, including the days, times subjects, etc., that the new person would cover. John accepted the changes and whenever he asked any questions relating to the subject the paper was added to or referred to.

Guided choices

Some children with autism need to be supported in making their own decisions in accepting changes or transitions.

Jonathan was motivated to finish his work because he knew that he was allowed to draw afterwards. However, he then found it hard to return to working again. Visual and verbal warnings were tried, but Jonathan was still unable to leave his activity. He was given written options to choose from, as shown in Figure 3, so that he had some ownership over his guided decision.

Once he had ticked his choice he set the timer. There were occasionally times when he did not automatically go when the bell rang, but instead of the teaching assistant having to get into discussion and disagreement with Jonathan she could just point to his recorded choice as a reminder.

As with all visual tools it is important that teachers and TAs design them, and use them, so they provide opportunities for us to use them flexibly. Leaving spaces which can be filled in with different information each time means that a pupil with autism is being taught to continue seeking information and to be adaptable to what that information says, within a clear and familiar structure.

Tick (✓) your choice and set the timer to the time you have chosen:

■ I will leave my drawing activity in **1 minute** and go to **lunch** …

■ I will leave my drawing activity in **4 minutes** and go to **lunch** …

When … the timer finishes … I will check my timetable or go to the next activity.

Figure 3 Written options for Jonathan to choose from

Tick (✓) your choice ....

■ I will leave my .... activity in ....

   minutes and go to ....

■ I will leave my .... activity in ....

   minutes and go to ....

When .... I will .... check

my timetable or go to the next activity.

The example card (Figure 3) was assessed for use initially just as a handwritten card. When this handwritten information was seen to be helpful to Jonathan in preparing for the transition time from his relaxing activity, it was made into a more substantial and flexible visual tool for long-term use. The card was laminated with a clear space for staff to write in the number of minutes that were guided choices and the next activity to go to. As these details were always different but set within a consistent framework, it meant that Jonathan had to really take notice of it and rigidity was carefully handled.

The card (page 59) can be photocopied and laminated. It can be used with a timer or without, depending on the pupil and the situation.

Social stories

Other students find social stories or power cards a useful way of gaining social information from which to make changes to behaviour or understand factors which help prevent anxieties and provide instructions in an easy-to-follow format.

Social stories, created by Carol Gray, are now a tool used regularly in many schools when catering for children on the autism spectrum.

Social stories are written in the first person as if the child has written it and provide an overall idea of what happens in situations and why, as well as what the child may need to do in such situations. Sentences are written to describe situations clearly, or to show what others might be thinking or feeling in the situation, and also sentences which suggest ways in which the child might try to do or say things. Social stories can be a useful strategy enabling children to prepare for forthcoming changes in the school context.

The social story opposite was written collaboratively by a Communication and Interaction team supporting a Year 4 pupil who was having difficulty listening to instructions in the classroom. The story was used to help him understand more fully what was being expected in class and how to change his behaviour so that he listened to what he was being asked to do.

Power cards are another very useful tool for teachers and TAs. Created by Elisa Gagnon, power cards use a child's special interest to help him gain an understanding of what he needs to do in a particular situation. Stories are created from the perspective of a hero or authority figure the child is very interested in. From this perspective some children feel very positive about the choices guided by their 'hero' figure and are able to remember what to do when a change in behaviour is required.

Jane, a pupil with autism, found it difficult to know when to ask questions or say things in class. Jane often talked about a variety of cartoon figures. A social story was written from the perspective of a favourite cartoon figure who described how 'he' knew when to speak in class and how to do it. A subsequent power card with the essential guidance points was created as a portable reminder for Jane. An example card is shown on page 62 which can be photocopied and adapted for children who are having this difficulty, using the name and picture of a favourite hero figure.

LISTENING TO MY TEACHER

There are many children in my class.

The teacher often talks to the whole class, giving information and instructions. Children in the class sit still and listen quietly while the teacher is talking.

I will try to sit still and listen quietly while the teacher is talking. Children in the class listen carefully to all the instructions and wait until the teacher asks them to start their work. The children know that if they start writing before they have heard all the instructions they may get the work wrong and have to do it again.

I will try to listen to all the instructions before starting my work, so that I have the best chance of getting it right the first time.

WAIT

The teacher will be very pleased with me if I sit still, listen well and wait to start my work until I am asked.

GO

Jane enjoyed the advice from the cartoon character, and was very willing to practise the steps to remember. They were acted out in a one-to-one session so that each part was understood. Once she was familiarized with what was expected the card was then used regularly in class. It is important to use help children use their reminder cards not only by using them *prior to situations* in which they may need them so as to prevent the difficulty occurring but also by *pointing to the relevant* words *immediately* the child begins to call out, so he recalls what to do without requiring verbal direction.

PICTURE OF HERO FIGURE

.... says 'Try to be like me when you want to speak in class.'

■ Put your hand up in the air and keep it there.

■ Wait quietly, without speaking.

■ A teacher will then ask you what you want to say.

■ Put your hand down and speak to the teacher.

■ Use a talking voice.

Sometimes challenging behaviour results in situations where children are stressed by changes and transitions. Chapter 5 considers some of the other reasons for challenging behaviour and further ways of supporting children in responding in new ways. If as teachers and TAs we consider how we can use good routines, familiarize children, use their special interests and guide them with good visual information we can sometimes prevent a build-up of anxiety and stress over changes and transitions for children on the autism spectrum.

Suggestions for helping children with autism to learn

MAKING SENSE OF CHANGES AND TRANSITIONS

- Understand the range of ways that children on the autism spectrum may perceive and respond to changes and transitions.

- Use routines and familiarization as ways of helping to decrease stress and teach new skills and behaviour.

- Use a range of other visual tools for teaching children on the spectrum to understand transitions and changes and to know what to focus on doing or saying in a range of situations.

- Refer to Chapters 4 and 5 to consider other ways of helping children to understand and accept changes and transitions and to be able to behave appropriately in different situations.

FURTHER READING

- Gagnon, E. (2006) *Power Cards. Using Special Interests to Motivate Children and Youth with Asperger Syndrome and Autism.* Shawnee Mission KS: Autism Asperger Publishing.

- Ling, J. (2006) *I can't do that. My Social Stories to help with Communication, Self-care and Personal Skills.* London: Paul Chapman.

- Shimmin, S. and White, H. (2006) *Every Day a Good Day. Establishing Routines in your Early Years Setting.* London: Paul Chapman.

Structuring a Meaningful Classroom

This chapter looks at what we mean by the components of structured teaching and visual approaches and how they can help teachers and TAs make the classroom make sense for children on the autism spectrum. The chapter considers:

- The principles behind structured teaching.

- Independence as a goal and its place in monitoring success.

- Making the *physical classroom environment* make sense.

- Making the *class timetable, routines and expectations* make sense.

- Making *lessons, activities and learning tasks* make sense.

Some children on the autism spectrum encounter numerous difficulties in school because they are unable to navigate either socially or organizationally what is expected of them in the classroom. This chapter focuses on what we mean by structured teaching and how this approach gives teachers the professional skills they need to help make the organization of the classroom make sense. It will consider how teachers can make small adjustments to enable individual pupils on the spectrum to more fully understand classroom expectations and to gain essential information which helps them to feel relaxed and able to learn.

The elements of structured teaching in this chapter are not new developments. Structured teaching is an important part of the TEACCH approach (Treatment and Education of Autistic and Communication-handicapped Children) and has been developed since the 1970s. TEACCH principles and elements of structured teaching and visual approaches are already used in many schools around the world to support the way that children on the autism spectrum learn. This chapter, along with some of the questions and answers in Chapter 6, recognizes the role that structured teaching already plays and considers how some myths and misconceptions have arisen in implementing structured teaching in practice. The chapter also suggests ways that teachers and teaching assistants can deepen their knowledge of how to use structured teaching so that individualization of these methods and the goal of independence for pupils become central to their success.

Structured teaching

Planning to meet the learning needs of a child on the autism spectrum requires teachers and teaching assistants to differentiate in the same way that they do for other children they teach. One of the simplest ways of differentiating is to ensure that the learning environments, activities, class or school routines all have the level of structure that each individual child on the autism spectrum needs to understand the expectations being placed upon them. Structured teaching means that teachers and teaching assistants prepare and organize themselves to present information, routines and learning in a way that enables the child to access them independently.

Structured teaching aims to help each pupil with autism receive the right level of structure. The right level being that which facilitates his independence. Structure aims to support difficulties with organization and comprehension, as well as prevent anxieties over misunderstanding information. Structure gives pupils safe learning environments from which to demonstrate their skills and knowledge.

From the teacher's or teaching assistant's perspective using the components of structured teaching enables them to plan effectively for a child or class. Below are the questions that teachers and TAs need to ask to help a pupil with autism learn and which identify the key components of the structured teaching approach.

- Is the learning environment helping a pupil to be focused on his learning? (Physical structure.)

- How does the pupil know where he has to go and when? (Timetable.)

- How does he know what he has to do there? (Work/activity instructions and systems.)

- How independent is the pupil able to be when participating in activities and lessons? (Visually clear tasks.)

In addition to these components of the structured teaching approach, teachers and teaching assistants also need to refine their skills in using these systems to ensure that they help a pupil with being adaptable. Teachers and TAs have to continually ask themselves:

- Are we using these systems to increase a child's flexibility? (Flexible factors.)

In order to simplify our thinking still further we can consider our planning questions from the child's perspective. What does the child we are working with want to know from us that may not be as obvious to him as it is to his peers?

- Where am I going?

- What do I have to do?

- How much am I expected to do?

- What will I do after I've finished this work?

One of the myths of using structured teaching is that it is time-consuming in terms of planning. It does sometimes take more preparation time to set up systems but the independence levels and success of pupils when these systems are in place are often worth the effort and the time spent decreases once good systems are in place. It is also important that we do not expect to do everything at once. Structured teaching is about using a clear process, moving step by step towards improved levels of focused and independent learning. The teaching process we use should enable us to target next steps and do so within a realistic framework. The framework suggests that teachers and TAs introduce small adjustments towards structuring for independence and when doing this we should expect to just produce basic tools initially to test out how effective they seem to be. Once we know they work this is the time to produce quality visual tools that can have long-term use. This way we do not waste time producing structures that are not yet right for a child.

Getting to know each pupil's learning strengths and difficulties and making small adjustments towards independence then is part of a teaching process. Structured teaching requires teachers and TAs to observe and assess where a child is having particular difficulties with learning, then to implement some levels of structure followed by a process of reassessment and restructuring (see Figure 4 opposite).

The measurement of success is simply that the child is able to learn or behave and is doing so as independently as possible. When observing and assessing teachers and teaching assistants are looking to see that a child understands *where* he needs to be, *what* work he is being asked to do, and *how* that work will be engaged with and completed and what will happen on completion.

For teachers and teaching assistants who believe in using structured teaching the initial goal is to make learning accessible through using visual timetables, visual activity work systems and other visual tools as a prerequisite to any other components of learning. Teachers and teaching assistants often cater for a wide range of needs in the classroom and are used to making adaptations and using special approaches to help children who are hearing-impaired, visually impaired, etc. For children on the autism spectrum the use of structure through visual systems can be just as necessary.

Teaching children on the autism spectrum can be tiring and time-consuming because the adaptations they often need require teachers and teaching assistant to spend time observing and structuring elements of the school day which other children do naturally. Some pupils on the autism spectrum may follow what is expected when told what to do and may exhibit no particular behaviour difficulties. Teachers and TAs sometimes comment that the pupil they work with is working well with their usual guidance and support and so

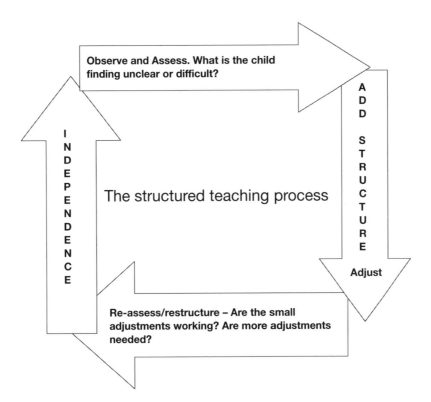

Figure 4 The structured teaching process

does not require any visual instructions or supports of any kind. Another misconception about the use of structure and visual tools is that they are not just necessary for managing behaviour or helping children who are not learning. These systems also help provide pupils with a way of receiving information which they can act upon independently without requiring verbal prompts. Teaching a pupil with autism to work, or move through the day by following visual instructions, is an important lifelong skill.

The goal of independence

One of the most rewarding elements of using structured teaching can be to see children experience the dignity of independence in how they carry out activities and participate in class routines. Assessing, structuring and restructuring routines and activities can be difficult to maintain amidst all the other challenges of working in a classroom but when students on the autism spectrum show that they can move around the classroom or school independently, follow their visual schedules and activity work systems independently and function as their peers are doing, teachers and teaching assistants can see clearly that the planning and preparation to enable this are worth doing.

It is important to not misunderstand the use of schedules or activity systems or other visual tools as simply aids to support what we instruct children to do. Sometimes they can be used in this way but if we remain using them only in this way then we are not using them to their full potential. The long-term goal in terms of using structure to support learning is for teachers and teaching assistants to set up the pupil's work and systems so effectively in terms of visual instructions that our role is unnecessary beyond the preparation and assessment. Progress can be measured by the child's level of independent functioning in the classroom.

Often teachers and teaching assistants are concerned about moving a child from objects to photographs, or photographs to symbols, or symbols to written levels of information giving. Sometimes it is helpful for a child to move to another level of receiving information. However, sometimes we are over-concerned with this and less concerned about establishing full independence. For example if the type of visual cue is changed from objects to photos, or from photos to symbols, and the child is less independent then the decision may not be beneficial for the child.

Teachers and teaching assistants need to think carefully about how a child demonstrates independence. If a child pulls a picture from his schedule or marks the next activity on his written schedule this may tell us only that he knows the routine and sequence of his schedule, not the meaning. Whereas if a child takes an art picture from his schedule, or ticks the word 'art' on his written schedule and without adult prompting goes to the art area, then we can see him demonstrate that the picture or word being used is meaningful to him and the level of visual cue being used is right for him with that activity.

Sometimes people ask, 'Should I go down a level, then?' when what they really mean is that we need to find the right level for the child. The 'right level' for each child means that the child can be independent in operating his systems and moving to and from activities or lessons without adult prompting. If a child is not independent, it is vital to find ways of making this happen. Sometimes a more able child can be more dependent than a less able child if he is not given the right level of visual support to enable him to be independent.

When a visual timetable, an activity or a routine is adjusted to improve upon it a pupil may react immediately by becoming more independent with that system and understanding it more easily. Sometimes we need to teach the child what we expect from any change we make and give him time to become accustomed to the restructuring. There are some children, however, who require a few days to accept a change in the system, even one that will be clearer for them eventually, and they require a short while to be taught and feel comfortable with the new aspects. Usually small adjustments to visual timetables or classroom systems do not take very long for the child to manage if they are presented at the right level. Even children with severe autism and other learning difficulties will respond quickly, within a few days, if our adjustments are right.

The three steps below help teachers and TAs to follow a process towards structuring for independence.

- Initially teachers and TAs need to assess and *teach each step* when first familiarizing a pupil with new work or new systems of working. However, it is important to be observant and to let a pupil do any aspects which he can without help. Good teaching with children on the autism spectrum is as much about knowing when not to intervene or communicate as about knowing when intervention is necessary to prevent a child getting something wrong.

- *Add structure to the activity* so that next time the steps that were too difficult can be done independently by the child.

- *Restructure* again if necessary and simplify for the child to be able to be independent and achieve success.

One of the important measures of success can be how little a teacher or teaching assistant needs to do or say for the child to be independent in carrying out a task.

It is not wrong for a child on the autism spectrum to follow verbal directions in the classroom, as that is part of classroom life. However, it is important to balance our thinking, as if the child is told on the spot what to do he will always expect to be told what to do and have no other system to rely on. This leaves some children unable to function without being told each step of what to do because they have become prompt-dependent.

Creating and using meaningful physical environments for learning

Physical structure refers to the way that furniture is arranged by teachers and TAs to give pupils helpful clues about where they are to sit or stand for an activity. Physical structure aims to clarify boundaries, minimize distractions and enable a child on the autism spectrum to be clear about expectations and be independent in using an area. Clear learning environments are helpful to all pupils, but with children on the autism spectrum it is even more important to define our classrooms or working areas so that a pupil does not misread situations and become distracted. It can be difficult for teachers and TAs to consider how differently some pupils with autism may think about furniture and room arrangements from pupils who are not on the spectrum. Sometimes an unclear learning environment can be the cause of a child on the spectrum displaying problematic behaviour. Considering how we use areas and give children clear signals in terms of physical structure is well worth reflecting upon.

CASE STUDY : SIMON

Simon, a Year 4 pupil in a special school, sometimes displayed difficulties when children moved to and from group sessions. A key problem was that whenever a few pupils were directed to leave the larger group to go to another working area, Simon would leap up and sit in each child's empty chair. When told not to, Simon took no notice at all and continued getting up and sitting down in every available chair.

What might staff think the behaviour was about?
It could have appeared to staff that Simon was unwilling to sit and wait while children were allocated to their work areas and became disruptive.

What else could it be?
When the teacher and TAs discussed the situation they realized that once all the chairs were removed from the seating area and put back around a table, Simon calmed down and was able to focus on his next activity. This helped staff to see that Simon was not being deliberately difficult but he was insecure about what the empty chairs next to him meant, and was unable to focus while they remained unused.

How did autism affect his behaviour?
Looking at this situation from Simon's perspective as a child with autism, the staff understood that once chairs were left empty Simon felt he had to sit in them and fill the space that was left. Simon may also have been unsure of where exactly he should be when others around him where moving and was also unable to concentrate because he did not have closure on the previous activity and a distinct start for the next one.

What did staff do to help?
To try and resolve this behaviour, pupils leaving the larger group were asked to take their chairs back to their tables before proceeding to the next activity or work area. This meant that there were no unoccupied chairs left standing about. Simon and the remaining children were encouraged to move their chairs in closer, then remain seated, waiting calmly for the smaller group session to start.

This example highlights how furniture without definite and meaningful functions can cause some pupils on the autism spectrum to feel unsure of what they do in an area. Considering how we position and arrange furniture can help a child know what is expected of him or her in a learning situation.

For some younger children in primary classrooms, early years settings, or those who are developmentally young and learn in special school classrooms (e.g. SLD), the way the classroom is arranged can be vital in helping them to gain clues as to what is expected of them. Some classrooms are small and where space is an issue some areas need to be used in a number of ways, for example a central table may have to function as a snack area and an activities area. Teachers need to help such areas look and operate differently to help them be clearly defined for the child and the purpose of the area visually understandable. In classrooms where there is limited space and dual uses for teaching areas, help pupils on the autism spectrum to be clear about the expectations of areas by using one of the following:

- Using different table coverings to depict different activities.

- Having place settings with the child's name or photograph.

- Having the children bring appropriate materials with them to the area as additional clues.

For pupils who can read, put written labels or signs on the table to remind them of their use, so that they can move from a written timetable to the designated place without verbal support.

Applying the principles of physical structure in the school or classroom involves considering all features of the learning environment and reducing those that might divert pupils from concentrating. Sometimes the environment we are using to teach children in does not take account of sensory discomfort or sensory overload for individual pupils. A child who has sensory problems with regulating his temperature may be sat near a radiator and may become very hot but be unable to convey this. Jackie, a pupil in a special class, would try to sit or stand against a radiator and did not move even though she was burning her skin. Other pupils can find it difficult to work under strip lighting, or to be where doors are opening and closing, or where too many people are passing behind them or next to noisy computers.

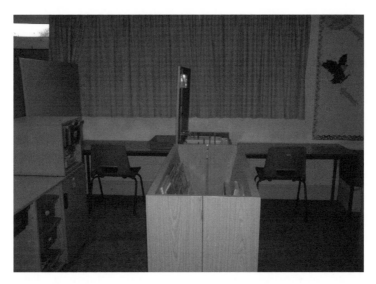

Figure 5 Where two pupils sit who require minimal distraction

Figure 5 shows where two pupils sit who require minimal distractions when working. To reduce sensitivity to light for these children a curtain is drawn. One of the two pupils likes to walk around when he has finished. The bookcase can be opened across his area, forming an easy boundary to allow him to move around without distracting other children who may be still working. The child who sits on the right requires space for his work activities to be put out on his left, organized along the shelf in a top-to-bottom formation. The child who sits on the left can collect his work activities from a tray and take them to his work desk so he requires a smaller work table area.

TRY THIS!

For children who can read and have moved to a new classroom try familiarizing them with where they are expected to work in this new setting. First write out and Blu-tack around the classroom the names of areas where they will be expected to go and work. Direct pupils to these by writing them on their timetables, e.g.:

Jason's timetable

- Jason's table – writing sheet 1.
- Book corner – sit and look at books until the teacher says it is group time.

Teach the child to follow these directions, looking for where he has to go and finding the area by reading the sign. If he finds such handwritten labels useful it is worth spending more time on making clear signs to help the pupil. Type out the classroom area names, laminate them and put them up. Use this method whenever the pupil has to work in a new room, area, etc.

For pupils who are able to read, labelling classroom areas can help them to be independent in going to the place indicated on their timetable.

For children who can read their timetable arrangements and find named areas, it can be a good idea to ensure that we do not make our written directions too rigid by making activities happen always in the same place. When this occurs our written timetable information becomes less necessary and the child can rely upon his visual memory of where he last did the activity or where he always does it. Whereas if a child can learn that he goes to the teacher table to do his next piece of work, and he has to look at where this is positioned each time, we are teaching him to be flexible and to scan his surroundings for visual clues. Enabling those children who are able to follow written directions to find areas that are labelled can maximize their learning.

The room area labels in Figure 6 can be photocopied, laminated and put up in different places for those children for whom this is the right level of information. They can be particularly useful when a child transitions to a new classroom where he may not be sure what activities go on in which place and where he needs to sit or go to for different activities. The labels in Figure 6 are just examples and can be adapted to meet the particular needs of each classroom and age range of children.

Calm Area

Teacher

Table

Book Corner

....'s

Table

Group Table 1

Figure 6 Room area labels

Helping Children with Autistic Spectrum Disorders to Learn, Paul Chapman Publishing © Mary Pittman 2007

For older and high-functioning students on the autism spectrum labels are helpful in relation to understanding where they are to sit and recognizing that they too may find their learning interrupted if they have difficulties with an overload of any sensory stimulation. Some students find themselves sitting under lights, or next to windows, or in the middle of the room, and dislike other children or adults walking behind them.

EXERCISE

What classroom areas do you need?

Think about all the activities and ways of working that you want to use in your classroom and consider how you have created or could create clear physical conditions which help the pupils with autism understand the context more clearly.

- A specific working area for each child – an independent work area, a desk, or a shared independent work area?

- A specific one-to-one working area for a child or a shared one-to-one work area which is timetabled?

- A whole-class work area – with seating arranged to maximize.

- A small-group work area – or more than one small group area.

- A play or leisure area – shared or individual.

- A calm area – shared or individual.

- A snack area.

As you consider the needs of the whole class along with the particular needs of children with autism the audit on page 75 could be used to help consider individual needs. The audit aims to help you determine which pupils on the autism spectrum are flexible in terms of where they sit and require no specific boundaries to help concentration, or any special requirements in terms of auditory, or visual stimulation.

Creating and using a meaningful timetable

A timetable or schedule is a visual means of a pupil knowing *where* he has to go for lessons or activities and the *order* in which he needs to go there.

There are many myths and misunderstandings about using timetables with children on the autism spectrum. When time is taken to look at what a timetable offers a child, where small adjustments could make them more meaningful and how they can be used in the classroom to help a pupil be more flexible, then they are likely to be of significantly more value.

Audit of the school/classroom environment

Use a highlighter pen to pinpoint where and how you could physically structure the learning environment differently for a pupil; or use it to identify where you already have established a good physical structure, which could be helpful information for other colleagues.

Feature	Level of current or potential intervention
Seating arrangements	■ Pupil is flexible in where he/she sits for every lesson or activity and displays no behaviours or anxieties related to his seating place but requires verbal direction where to sit.
	■ Pupil could/does benefit from a designated place to sit for each lesson or activity.
	■ Pupil could/does benefit from a level of seating boundary to minimize distractions, e.g. position of table and chair facing the wall, or use of a portable screen or curtained area.
	■ Pupil could/does benefit from seating areas to move to in the classroom which designate working arrangement and are used only for a set purpose, e.g. independent workstation or desk, one-to-one working table, group table, whole-class seat and table.
	■ Pupil could/does benefit from moving his own chair to and from different areas as a means of individually structuring classroom movement to areas.
	■ Pupil could/does benefit from an independent working base as his main seating place, with movement to and from that booth for specific lesson activity only.
Calm areas	■ Pupil could/does benefit from time using a specified calm area of the classroom or school and can take himself there as needed.
	■ Pupil could/does benefit from regular direction from staff to move to a specified calm area of the classroom.
	■ Pupil could/does benefit from regular timetabled use of a specified calm area for short periods.
	■ Pupil could/does benefit from spending more extensive time in a specified calm area for parts of the day or week known to be problematic.
Areas to use in break or lunchtime	■ Pupil could/does benefit from a being directed to specific areas of the playground, e.g. swing, sand area, quiet seat, through a mini-schedule.
	■ Pupil could/ does benefit from using a special-interest activity during break time.
	■ Pupil could/does benefit from using a break-time quiet area, a special break-time club, a peer/buddy system during break or lunchtime.
Sensory considerations	Consider any features of the learning environment that cause the pupil difficulties with sensory overload, e.g.:
	■ Strip lights.
	■ Windows.
	■ Computer screens.
	■ Noisy equipment.
	■ Noisy peers.
	■ Next to a radiator.

A timetable can be used to give pupils with autism a range of useful information which they often do not easily have access to, unless they are relying on their visual memory, which when plans change is not possible to do. A timetable broadly offers a child information about:

■ Where they are going or what is happening *now*.

■ What is going to happen in the *future*.

■ When an activity *starts* and *finishes*.

■ When *something different* is going to occur.

Timetable information needs to be offered at a meaningful level. A test of 'meaningful' is that a child quickly learns to look at the information being presented and go to the place independently, as directed by the visual information and not by any verbal or other cues.

Information can be presented at a number of levels and it is important to use the level which a pupil can understand and follow, even on a day when he is feeling stressed and upset. This often means presenting information at a level which is easier for the child, and at his comfort level rather than his challenge level. Information can be presented by using:

■ Objects.

■ Photographs.

■ Pictures.

■ Icons/symbols.

■ Written formats.

Children with autism, like other children, will need to make judgements about sequences of events and time. These judgements include when things are to happen, the order of events, how long the children will be doing something for, when it actually starts, when it finishes, whether it is the same order as usual or a different order. Depending upon age and developmental level, pupils may need to focus on:

■ The immediate.

■ First-and-then sequences.

■ Half-day sequences.

■ Whole-day sequences.

Other pupils may also require some judgements about whole weeks or even months in certain circumstances.

When using a timetable teachers and TAs need to ensure that its visual presentation, the style of information and the time sequencing and the level of involvement of the child are all matched correctly to his individual understanding level.

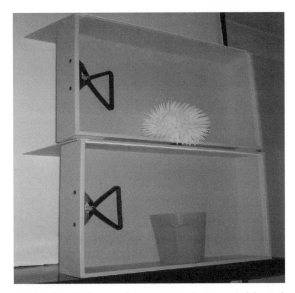

Figure 7 A simple first – then, top-to-bottom object timetable

Figure 7, shows a simple first-and-then, top-to-bottom, object timetable. This format was used with Simon, a boy who could collect his next timetable object himself if his system was set out clearly. Simon liked to know what was happening next but found it difficult to absorb too much information. The objects in the photograph are a sensory ball indicating the play area and his cup, depicting drink/snack time. The 'timetable' was made by placing two box files on top of each other fastened together using Velcro.

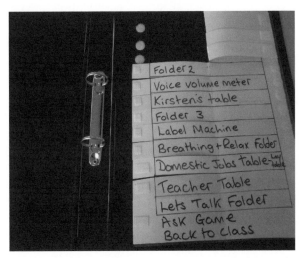

Figure 8 A timetable written on laminated card with a wipe-off pen

Figure 8 shows a timetable written on laminated card with a wipe-off pen. The timetable is set into an ordinary file folder for portable use. Rachel, a student with autism and moderate learning difficulties, refused to put a tick or draw a line through to indicate her progress. After some assessment and discussion with Rachel, the timetable was cut into sections and she folded each activity across and attached it with Velcro to show progress through the day. The timetable was written in two colours: one depicted where the student was going, e.g. to the teacher's work table, to a peer's work table, to another room or area, and then in a different colour what the pupil would do in each area was indicated where appropriate.

77

Audit of timetable structures

Feature	Level of current or potential intervention
Time perspective	Pupil does/could benefit from: ■ A weekly or termly school timetable with highlighted areas and extra information about rules to remember. ■ A daily timetable co-ordinated to school bell times referred to through the day. ■ A whole-day activity sequenced timetable. ■ A half-day activity sequenced timetable. ■ A first-and-then-style sequenced timetable. ■ A visual cue given immediately prior to the event. ■ A timetable related to changeable home events such as respite care days, weekends etc.
Style of visual information for the timetable	Pupil does/could benefit from a timetable that is presented in the following form or combination of forms to provide easily accessible information: ■ real objects ■ symbolic objects ■ photographs ■ icons (colour picture images) ■ symbols (line drawn black and white) ■ written ■ a combination of styles, e.g. icons for some areas and photos for others, written with symbols for one or two areas, etc.
Presentation *Individual timetables*	Pupil does/could benefit from the daily timetable being presented for individual use: ■ In a wallet or diary. ■ In a book or folder. ■ Attached to a clipboard. ■ On a laminated board.
Class timetable	Pupil does/could benefit from the daily timetable being presented for the whole class: ■ Written on a whiteboard for sporadic reference or benefits from teacher/TA making direct reference to it through the day to start and end lessons. ■ Presented as a symbol/picture timetable with teachers or teaching assistants making reference to the timetable to start and end lessons and /or involving pupils in operating the class timetable.
Features	Pupil does/could benefit from the daily timetable having features such as: ■ A way of distinguishing the current activity from those still to come, e.g. a 'time for' box. ■ A way of depicting that an activity/lesson has finished, e.g. a pencil line through the activity, a tick box, a finished or 'all done' pocket. ■ Clarification of words which have more than one meaning, e.g. PE may mean large apparatus or small apparatus, Art may mean drawing or painting, etc. ■ Clarification of activities or lessons by focusing on a different aspect, e.g. does the pupil need to know *what* he is to be doing, or does he feel knowing *where* he is to go for the activity is more important, or does he need to know *who* he is to be working with to make the information more understandable?
Location	Pupil does/could benefit from the timetable being physically accessible, e.g.: ■ Hung on a board near the individual student's work area. ■ Placed on a desk or table. ■ Portable and carried around in a pocket, file, folder, book, wallet, etc.

STRUCTURING A MEANINGFUL CLASSROOM

Use the audit on page 68 to consider where and how you could use a timetable format with a pupil with autism, or where you could further develop one or two attributes of its use.

Using work or activity systems

There are a number of ways in which systems can be set up for pupils to carry out independent work, leisure activities, daily living tasks, etc. This chapter is not considering activity systems in the wider sense but concentrating on how independent work can be organized and used in the classroom.

Enabling a child to do some activities independently whereby established skills are practised can be very useful in any classroom setting. Establishing ways in which a pupil can do independent work is a component of structured teaching which can be used flexibly to help a pupil in parts of the day or parts of a lesson where he is finding it difficult to participate. Some children with autism enjoy their working times in the classroom but find any unstructured elements difficult, and again independent work sessions can then be very useful, enabling the child to feel pleased with his success in practising existing skills and also feeling clear about what he can do in a less structured period of time. When a child is in a working situation he needs a clear system which clarifies for him:

- What work to do.

- The amount of work to do.

- A way of judging progress.

- What will happen afterwards.

These questions apply to independent work settings and also to any lesson. Sometimes children in group-work situations or whole-class lessons also need these same questions answered for them through a clear system. Work systems, as with other visual tools, are a way to help a child know what he has to do without relying on his visual memory, which may mean the child tries to be rigid in his working practices.

For some children work activities need to be presented on the child's left, in a linear arrangement that clearly shows how many tasks are ready for him to do. On the child's right there will be a container in which the child can place his completed work. Following the work activities there needs to be something which helps a child to know what he is doing next – either returning to his timetable or going immediately to a favourite activity.

Other children can follow a set of visual instructions which let him know to collect each activity in a work tray or basket. For example, a child may have an activity strip with a shape on it which he can collect and match to a basket with the same shape on it indicating this is the basket of work he needs to take to his work desk. Children who have a strength or interest in 'matching' find these forms of work systems useful.

Other pupils can use work systems which are written directions to collect colour files from a hanging-file folder system as in Figures 9 and 10. Consider the variety of ways that work systems could be established or are being established on the audit. There may be other formats as well as those listed.

WORK TO DO

Red file folder _ ✓

Yellow file folder _

Check timetable

Figure 9 A linear arrangement that clearly shows how many tasks are ready to do

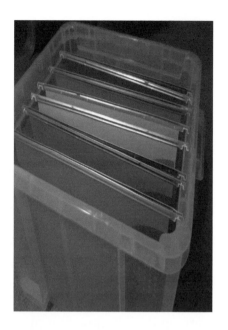

Figure 10 Work systems can be contained in hanging file folders, colour-coded

Making sense of tasks

As well as considering how work or activity systems help a child understand what to do, it is also important that any activities the child is to do are clearly structured. The tasks should be achievable independently without any help from a teacher or TA. If the activities cannot be done correctly or the child needs help to do them, they are not useful as part of an independent work system until practised through one-to-one teaching.

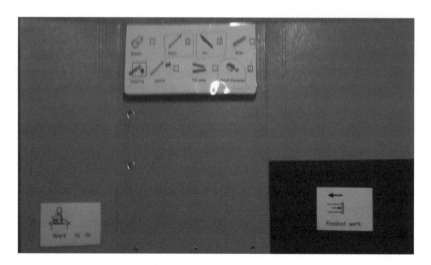

Figure 11 A folder used to help a pupil to be more independent in collecting resources

The folder shown in Figure 11 is used to help a pupil to be more independent in collecting the resources he needs to do a worksheet. A worksheet can be positioned under the fold-down flap with pictures or symbols of materials that the student may require. In the left pocket a simple instruction card can be placed, reminding the student to collect the equipment he needs. The student himself or a teacher/TA can using a wipe-off pen,

80

Audit for independent work systems

Feature	Level of current or potential intervention (highlight)
Visual instructions for work system	Pupil does/could benefit from: ■ Written 'to do' list of folders to work from. ■ Shapes, colours, numbers, letters to remove and match. ■ Pictures related to a special interest to remove and match. ■ Tasks set out in a linear arrangement (top to bottom or left to right).
Style of work system	Pupil does/ could benefit from: ■ An independent work file with dividers which present a 'work to do' section and a 'finished work' section, along with a set of instructions for using the file in flexible ways. ■ An independent work folder which opens to display a 'work to do' pocket and a 'finished work' pocket. ■ A hanging file folder system. ■ An independent work box or work tray with separate transparent wallets containing a range of practical tasks to be done. ■ Tasks presented without containers but with all parts of each task attached so that each one is self-contained.
Organization of work system	Folder contains written instructions on how much work to do and the pupil follows the written guidelines for a variety of situations. Folder contains flexible amounts of work which can be continued as needed or filed as unfinished and returned to as and when appropriate and self-managed by the pupil. Folder contains only work to be done at that time and is managed by a supporting adult. Pupil can follow flexible amounts of work by following whatever colour, shape or number card system is presented, e.g. tray 1, tray 2, tray 3. Work box or work tray contains only work to be done at that time and is managed by the adult.
Collection and/or placement of work system	■ Pupil carries from class to class one portable file/folder system containing independent worksheets and finished section. ■ Pupil carries a portable 'work to do' folder or file but requires two separate folders for finished work and/ or unfinished work. ■ Pupil goes to a central place in a classroom to collect a work box or tray and a 'finished tray'. ■ Pupil places the work box or work tray at appropriate working distances, with work to do on the left and the 'finished' box or tray on the right. ■ Pupil requires a card system for where to position 'work to do' box/tray and 'finished work' box/tray at the right distance. ■ Pupil requires adult to set out the work tasks for the pupil to do.
Content of work systems (ideas)	Pupil does/could benefit from: ■ Worksheets to practise existing skills in literacy, numeracy, science, ICT and other subject areas. ■ Workbooks or laminated worksheets from which to practise existing skills in various subject areas. ■ Handwriting practice sheets/colouring sheets. ■ Matching and sorting practice tasks relating to literacy, numeracy other subject areas. ■ Assembling tasks with pictures to demonstrate what to do. ■ Stacking, putting in, pulling apart tasks.

Helping Children with Autistic Spectrum Disorders to Learn, Paul Chapman Publishing © Mary Pittman 2007

encircle the items that the pupil needs to collect, e.g. pen, pencil, ruler, etc., and the pupil can tick these when he has collected them. This folder also allows a clear system of directing the pupil to put a finished worksheet into his 'finished work' pocket after completion.

For teachers and TAs working in special schools or those working in other settings where there are a number of pupils on the autism spectrum in one class, it can be difficult to design materials or tasks that will allow the assessment of different levels of ability.

The adapted book folder in Figure 12 demonstrates how teachers and teaching assistants can make a folder which is multi-purpose and can be used with a number of different children on the autism spectrum, operating at differing levels of reading or book accessibility. The folder format allows a variety of books to be attached, using Velcro, to an A3 central section of the folder. The space allows the book to be opened easily without obscuring the left-hand view. On the page or pages positioned on this end of the folder a teacher or TA can affix with Velcro words, symbols or pictures for a child to place to each page of the books as appropriate to their ability.

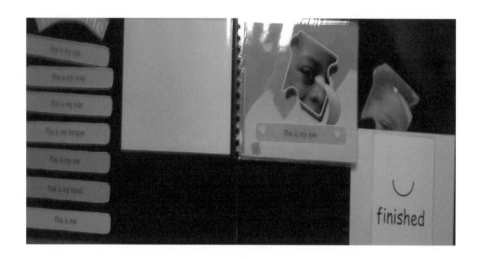

Figure 12 An adapted folder which is multi-purpose and can be used with a number of children

If a child is unable to operate at this level the left-hand section of the folder can be folded away. The book can then be organized with a right-hand side finished pocket so that a child may access the book by pulling off the key picture and placing it in the 'finished' pocket before turning to the next page. One folder can therefore, if designed and laminated carefully, be useful in a number of ways.

When working with younger children or children who require adaptation of books to access them it is often necessary to have several copies of a book so as to be able to rearrange or organize them so that they are sufficently differentiated.

There are many ways in which tasks can be adjusted so that activities are clearly understood and differentiated, and teachers and TAs find themselves producing these day by day. For further information on how to visually structure activities TEACCH have produced a series of books 'Tasks Galore' which provide a range of task examples for pupils of different ages and levels of ability. They are listed at the end of this chapter.

Other factors in the use of visual tools

Schools, departments, individual teachers and TAs need to consider their views on when, why and how visual approaches can be used to enable children to find their school lives more meaningful. Throughout this book there are references to the use of visual tools or visual supports and how writing things down or using pictures, objects or photographs are all ways of helping a child to see what is expected rather than having to process verbal information or 'read between the lines', both of which are particular difficulties for children with autism. Using written information, symbols, icons, photographs or objects to enable children to understand at the right level for each of them has to be worth teachers and TAs using as a communicative toolbox.

When using symbols, some schools or departments in schools believe that there should be one source of symbols used throughout the school with all the children who require them, so that there is consistency of approach. Other schools have pupils with such a range of severe or complex needs that individual pupils need very specific sources if the symbols are to be really effective and understood clearly, so an eclectic mix of symbol programmes is used, along with digital photographs, etc. The most important factor is that a child understands what we want from him, and school policies and practices need to agree upon and use the systems that provide a child with meaningful information. The section on useful web sites at the back of this book provide further information for schools or classes who want to consider the range of symbol options that exist.

The last audit in this chapter (page 84) refers to the use of other tools such as visual reminders, routines and rewards which can sometimes be helpful with individual pupils.

Flexibility factors

Sometimes teachers and TAs mistakenly believe that components of structured teaching from the TEACCH approach are likely to make children more rigid in their thinking. However, the whole principle of using structure and visual tools is to enable children on the autism spectrum to be more flexible. For example, whenever possible we need to consider if we are actively teaching flexibility in the way we use the components of structure or visual supports.

When using a timetable it is important to consider how we can teach a child to accept changes on it. For some children it may mean using a special 'surprise' symbol, for others it may mean putting a line through something and adding the alternative activity. As change is difficult for a child on the autism spectrum initially, we need to accustom such a child to the system we are going to use. It is important when first teaching these points to change an activity that the child is not so happy to do for one that he really is motivated to do. Equally, when providing independent work systems it is important to prevent a pupil from becoming rigid about the number of tasks or the order of tasks he is to do.

Sometimes teachers and TAs can spend considerable amounts of time individualizing arrangements so that a pupil can be more independent and less reliant on the teacher or TA to interpret in each situation what he has to do. Constant verbal prompting can result

Audit of visual reminders, routines, rewards

Features of visual tools	Level of current or potential intervention
Visual routines	■ Pupil does/could benefit from written routines which explain what happens and is expected at points in the day such as registration, breaks, lunchtimes, walking to and from playground, etc.
	■ Pupil does/could benefit from pictures/photographs which sequence a routine or routines, which happen in the school day.
	■ Pupil does/could benefit from a specific intervention in relation to one routine, e.g. visual registration board, a lining-up route designated, a knowledge of who is to be in charge of set jobs for the day, a visual turn-taking rota for clearing up or using the computer.
Visual rewards	■ Pupil does/could benefit from receiving tokens/points towards a reward and visual reminder(s) of what he has to do to attain these, referred to as each lesson starts.
	■ Pupil does/could benefit from a visual reward system based on a picture of a favourite activity or subject to talk about, divided into jigsaw pieces to be attained during the day during different lessons to earn time with that activity.
Visual reminders	■ Pupil can/does benefit from written reminders that are written and referred to daily, e.g. 'Raise hand and wait for the teacher to speak to you if you have a question or need some help.'
	■ Pupil can/does benefit from picture clues to remind him of behaviour expectations.

in less independence than the pupil is really capable of, and may sometimes even cause the child distress and confusion because he is having to process verbal instructions, or the lack of visual clarity is difficult for him to cope with. Once systems are in place the preparation work load does become easier, but the maintenance of these support systems such as timetables and work systems does to some degree still continue to demand energy, time and commitment if the pupil is to be successful. There is also the need to remind ourselves that any visual or organizational tools that are used in the classroom require those who plan and prepare them to think flexibly about how the pupil will use them. It can be all too easy in busy classrooms to allow visual and organizational tools like timetables or work systems to become so routine or unchanging that they became part of a child's rigidity rather than providing him with a means of flexibly coping.

The last exercise in this chapter provides a case study of a pupil with autism who is having quite extreme difficulties, This exercise could be used by individual teachers or TAs to help them reflect, or it could be used by staff teams to promote discussion and apply the principles of structured teaching.

Case study – staff development exercise

The case study below can be used as a staff development exercise to help teachers and teaching assistants consider how components of structure could be used to help a pupil overcome the anxieties and consequent behaviour difficulties which resulted in him failing to learn in a new setting. Read the case study introduction and then consider each component of the structured teaching approach and how it could be applied to Jason. A number of possible ways forward could be identified by staff doing this exercise. These could be compared with what the staff at Jason's school actually did to enable him to overcome his difficulties and learn.

INTRODUCING JASON

A Year 7 pupil, Jason was very unsettled by his move to secondary school and within weeks found himself unable to cope with going into the main school building, or being a member of his class. Owing to his extreme anxiety and confusion his behaviour became difficult and he would shout, hit or kick furniture over. Eventually the only way Jason could come to school was to work in a side room of the special needs learning resource base which had its own entrance and did not involve him having to use the main entrance. The room he was occupying with his TA was a small one with four tables in it and six chairs. Each day Jason came in and rearranged the furniture.

Jason's anxiety and consequent behaviour reached a high pitch and he was unable to do any school work at all. His mother was working hard to get him to attend but he would clearly have preferred not to. The only activities that Jason would do were; take a walk around the grounds when other pupils were working and were not around, read his comics, draw, and talk about woodland creatures or read books about them. He was refusing to do all formal school work and everything he did do was of his own choice. The staff at the school wondered whether Jason would be better placed in a special school. It was impossible at this stage to really see what skills he had because the confusion he felt masked them.

What would you do about Jason's difficulties?

After reading about Jason, carry out the following three exercises as you consider how the components of structured teaching could help Jason. Note that there may be more than one way to introduce good components of structure to support a pupil and, after you have considered what you would do, read what the staff at Jason's school did to enable him to reduce his anxieties and learn.

EXERCISE 1 USING PHYSICAL STRUCTURE WITH JASON

What might the first steps be in helping Jason to feel more settled with the physical structure of the room?

Staff considered that Jason felt he had to arrange the furniture because he was unsure of its purpose and this might have been stressful for him. The staff had to decide whether they should continue allowing him to arrange the furniture as he felt happier that way or should they arrange the furniture themselves so that it had clear functions? To make the room useful initially Jason required three areas, a one-to-one teaching area, an independent workplace and a snack/leisure table area. The one-to-one teaching area required two chairs, one for Jason and one for his TA. The independent workplace required just one chair for Jason; and for the leisure/snack area a small side table and an easy chair were positioned. Any additional chairs or tables were removed. Each of the three areas was labelled using words that Jason used himself or words he was aware of. His one-to-one teaching area was 'Mrs Smith's table' (his TA), his leisure area was referred to as 'Jason's reading place', and his own work table was recorded as 'Jason's table'. Immediately on entering the classroom Jason was told that the room was now arranged for him, and he was immediately directed to 'Jason's reading place', where one of his favourite comics was waiting for him.

EXERCISE 2 USING A TIMETABLE WITH JASON

What would a simple timetable look like for Jason?

After being given time to settle with his comic, Jason was given a simple written timetable that incorporated activities that he could tolerate without too much upset and he was given opportunities to move around the three areas as directed on the written timetable. These were later extended to include a short early visit to the school canteen, a trip to the library to go and pick up a favourite book and come out, etc. Initially his timetable read as a list and had no specific times on it; just a simple work-then-relax routine was put in place and even where he was expected to be at a work table the work was built around his interests until he began to be less stressed and showed this through his co-operation.

EXERCISE 3 ENGAGING JASON IN LEARNING

How could Jason be encouraged to start doing activities and developing a work ethic?

Initially all Jason's work focused around his favourite subject of woodland creatures. He wrote about them, researched them, drew them, etc. Gradually this took him to various parts of the school, for example to the library or computer suite, etc. As Jason settled over the next few weeks expectations were extended so that he did some curriculum work, followed by his special-interest work. His special-interest work gradually became his independent work and he followed a variety of work systems with this favourite subject.

Moving on with Jason

Starting at a very basic level with Jason allowed him to rebuild his confidence and to develop knowledge about his setting and what was expected of him. Once the timetable and work systems were taught to Jason he could then feel more secure about going into other settings. He was always given preparatory visits and small preparatory steps.

Gradually Jason accepted going to registration, to the canteen, into part of a lesson, and over the next year and a half he moved into being fully included as well as successful in a number of subject exams.

Setting up supportive information systems allows a child on the autism spectrum to make sense of what is expected. These systems enable a pupil to feel calm and able to demonstrate the skills he has. Using the components of structured teaching, teachers and teaching assistants provide pupils with support systems which can help them be included in a meaningful classroom environment.

Suggestions for helping children with autism to learn

STRUCTURING A MEANINGFUL CLASSROOM

- Assess and identify difficulties in learning or behaviour.
- Apply the principles and relevant components of structured teaching to enable the child to be more independent and successful.
- Plan and use visual systems in a way which teaches or maintains flexible thinking while using the components of structure.
- Pursue the goal of independence through visual structure.
- Refer to Chapter 6 to review some frequently asked questions relating to misconceptions and solutions in the use of structure to help children learn.

FURTHER READING

- Eckenrode, L., Fennell, P. and Hearsey, K. (2004) *Tasks Galore Early Education*. Raleigh, NC: Tasks Galore Publishing.

- Eckenrode, L., Fennell, P. and Hearsey, K. (2004) *Tasks Galore for the Real World*. Raleigh, NC: Tasks Galore Publishing.

- Mesibov, G. and Howley, M. (2003) *Accessing the Curriculum for Pupils with Autistic Spectrum Disorders. Using the TEACCH Programme to Help Inclusion*. London: David Fulton.

Behaviour: Simplifying the Problem-solving Process

This chapter looks at the way in which teachers and TAs can read the communicative messages which children on the autism spectrum present through the way they behave. It concentrates our thinking and planning on what we want the child to do rather than on what he is not doing, so that behaviour challenges can be resolved. The chapter is also concerned with how teachers and TAs support themselves and other colleagues as they work with children who are displaying behaviour challenges. The chapter focuses on;

- Defining what we mean by challenging behaviour.

- Understanding behaviour as communication.

- Simplifying our approach to solving behaviour challenges.

- Working together to successfully analyse challenging behaviour.

- Using a staged approach to problem solving such as SPACE in order to support both the pupil and the adults who are working with him.

Children on the autism spectrum do not always display challenging behaviour. However, they are often unable to communicate what they are thinking or feeling, cannot process and understand what is being asked of them, or read the relevant social messages. These communication difficulties can lead to feelings of confusion and anxiety, which leave the child using the only means of expression he has left, behaviour. Behaviour can therefore be a major indicator of how comprehensive our structures are and how comfortable a pupil with autism is feeling within our setting.

This chapter helps us to establish whether children are displaying behaviours which are situation-specific or behaviours which are more confusing, chaotic or random in presentation. Children who are frequently displaying challenging behaviour are making demands on their own coping reserves as well as often being demanding on the coping reserves of those around them too. Children with autism who are displaying challenging behaviour are unpredictable, and likely to be experiencing a cycle of stress which is difficult for them and for those around them. A child with structure and predictability, along with relaxation interspersed into his day, is more likely to unwind so that behaviour becomes more manageable and is more situation-specific rather than random and chaotic.

In some situations, staff may need to reorganize situations in order to establish new positive behaviours and routines which can replace those that have been problematic. With other children who have more understanding, the focus of strategies may need to be on teaching the child what is expected of him, through revealing information which previously was 'hidden' from the child's view of the world.

In addition to considering what is happening with the child, the chapter considers how challenging behaviour affects the professionals or adults who are supporting him. As part of our problem-solving process, it is vital that adults receive useful guidance which can help break any stress cycles. One of the approaches suggested in this chapter is to give ourselves and the child 'space' from the situation causing the behaviour difficulty while we readjust and replan, so that we clarify for the child what we want him to do. In this chapter using 'space' from a situation that we know is causing major upset, while we plan a different strategy is not considered an avoidance tactic but simply a temporary measure which prevents a child becoming set in a pattern of difficult responses that he can no longer control. In this chapter SPACE, an acronym (Stress, Prevention, Action, Calming Environments or Extras), provides us with an action planning tool for supporting pupils on the autism spectrum who are presenting challenging behaviour.

What do we mean by challenging behaviour?

When we consider that a child displays 'challenging behaviour' we can mean a range of different things. Challenging behaviour can be behaviour which causes distress to the child or those around him, or which directly or indirectly interferes with the child's learning and which reduces or restricts his long term opportunities. The word 'challenging' reminds us that those of us who work with children on the autism spectrum are challenged to solve the difficulty.

It is important that teachers and TAs and schools consider their beliefs about challenging behaviour when it is presented by a child with autism rather than by a child with a different diagnosed or undiagnosed difficulty. The definition of challenging behaviour may be the same, but the reasons for behaviour difficulties in children with autism, and usually the strategies which resolve them, require responses that are meaningful in terms of their autism.

The nature of autism makes it unlikely that a child will be able to change his actions himself, unless the adults who support him do something definite to alter the situation. Children on the autism spectrum are often powerless to change their behaviour and are reliant on the adults who work with them to initiate new responses or routines that enable them to act differently. With some pupils, to do this we need to give them the right information to know what they need to do; other pupils may need the environment or routines recreated so that they know what they are meant to do in a situation.

The term 'challenging behaviour' generally refers to behaviour which can:

- be frequent.

- be extreme.

- last a long time.

- be harmful to the child or others.

- prevent learning from taking place.

Challenging behaviour is often considered to result from a child not knowing how to gain attention, or because of a desire for control, among other factors.

However, when considering a child with autism, there is a need to consider that challenging behaviour may be occurring because of his autism, which leaves him:

- Unsure or unaware of what to do or say.

- In a set behaviour routine which he feels compelled to carry out.

How challenging is the challenging behaviour?

Some children on the autism spectrum present challenging behaviour which we can classify as 'situation-specific', in that it occurs only in set situations or circumstances, which we can clearly identify. Sometimes, however, we are working with autistic children who are displaying a more constant and chaotic pattern of challenging behaviour which has become difficult for us to predict.

Situation-specific behaviour challenges

If a pupil is displaying behaviour challenges in situation-specific settings, he is generally calm and learning well in other situations, while finding one specific lesson, activity or context difficult, or has one particular misunderstanding that he displays across contexts.

Teachers and TAs tend to feel confident that they can find a solution to a particular difficulty, as this is set among a number of other successes that the pupil is experiencing. Teachers and TAs learn from these situations and can often grow in confidence in their knowledge of the pupil and may be able to predict which situations may cause future difficulties for the child. Teachers, TAs and others who support the child are equipped to predict potential areas of difficulty and prepare the child for them, which is likely to reduce future behaviour difficulties.

The factors which cause situation-specific behaviour challenges can usually be identified by staff with a sound knowledge of autism. These can then be considered at a strategy level which matches the child's understanding in order to redirect or replace the behaviour.

Regular yet unpredictable incidents of challenging behaviour

By contrast, a pupil may present a number of challenging behaviours or the same challenging behaviour in many situations. This can be difficult for staff to cope with because the behaviours occur randomly and no two days feel the same. Consequently it is not easy to identify a pattern of behaviour. This can leave staff, parents and the child himself feeling confused, unable to identify where and when challenging behaviours are likely to happen and what impact they are having upon it.

When a pupil has become overwhelmed by his challenging behaviours in this way, he is unlikely to be able to display the skills he has, and is likely to considerably underperform. Teachers and TAs can be left feeling that there are very few parts of the day, if any, that are consistently successful for the child, and this can result in staff feeling deskilled and stressed, unable to break the cycle, in fact sometimes adding to the cycle of stress. When experiencing a bombardment of challenging behaviours, the child is in a more cumulative state of stress, which in turn compounds the problem.

Understanding behaviour as communication

Behaviour can be a key indicator of whether a child with autism is feeling calm and clear about what is expected of him. Behaviour difficulties are often the result of a child misunderstanding expectations or feeling unclear about what he is meant to do or say in a particular situation or may be the result of accumulative stress.

The child who is experiencing situation-specific behaviour challenges seems to be trying to tell us that 'Whenever I am in this situation I do not know what is expected of me, how to do or say what I am meant to, how long I will be here, etc. A pupil who is generally working well in school, but becomes negative or abusive when attending larger school occasions like assemblies, or when there are changes in the school programme of trips or special events, is displaying situation-specific behaviour.

A pupil who is generally working well in the classroom except in certain lessons, certain parts of the day, for instance lunch break, or when asked to work in certain contexts such as in groups, or is anxious about sitting near one particular pupil, is displaying behaviour which is situation or context-specific.

A child who is displaying regular yet unpredictable behaviour challenges seems to be trying to tell us that 'There are so many parts of my day that feel demanding or unclear that sometimes, just out of the blue, I cannot cope any longer.' Clearer routines, structures, relaxing activities and information are needed so that a child can function more consistently and find a coping level from which to recover from cumulative stress. Some pupils, however, come into school and it seems that staff are unsure how they will react in any part of the day or week and they may be reacting to cumulative stresses and confusion. These children are likely to need clearer and more defined structures throughout their day. The general communication from this child is that he is not happy or that he can become easily stressed and confused about what is expected of him. The more unpredictable the pupil's behaviour very often the more the child needs to be able to predict his environment and be successful and may need modifications to be made so that what he has to do is so obvious that he cannot get it wrong, which in turn will help him break the cycle. Often very tight and basic structures help a child back on the road to success quite quickly.

The list on pages 94–5, is not exhaustive, but contains a number of possible autism-related difficulties which could trigger a challenging behaviour response and a suggested communicative response that a child might give, if he were able to explain his behaviour. The list also suggests where we might be able to target our strategies to enable the child to overcome his behaviour difficulty. Cumulative stress, demand or sensory overload are factors which have a lot in common in triggering challenging behaviour responses from children with autism.

With cumulative stress it can be difficult for teachers, TAs or others to predict that a major upset is likely. Over time, adults often become used to any signals which pinpoint this. However, often a pupil moves rapidly from appearing calm and compliant to suddenly not coping at all. Sometimes parents report that their child comes home very difficult to manage while in school he has really not been any problem and is progressing at a good rate, in terms of school activities and expectations. It is easy to forget that as these children cannot recognize or self-regulate their own needs, they may not be able to give themselves time to relax unless we help them to organize it and specifically put relaxation times into their school day in order to avoid a build-up of stress. Equally, we need to communicate carefully with parents to see if there are any changes at home which the child is having to adjust to. If there are, sometimes the pupil experiences them as another demand on his coping reserves and we need to consider how we can help him find some extra relaxation or recovery time for a short while.

Demand overload can be closely linked with cumulative stress. Using the activity system structures discussed in the previous chapter, we can see how some children can feel overloaded by demands if we are not setting out clearly how much they have to do, or how long they will be in a teaching situation. If what we are expecting of a child is realistic in terms of the child's stress level, then being visually clear about how much work there is to do and being clear that there is something relaxing or motivating to do afterwards can be most helpful. However, if we are expecting more and more of a pupil and not monitoring how he is coping with it, and considering any other factors which may be causing him anxiety, then 'seeing' a lot of work to do may become a demand rather than a clear structure. This can also be true with timetables or any of the systems we are using. It does not mean that our systems are wrong in themselves, only that they may, at times, need adjusting for a pupil who is temporarily not coping well. If this is happening, we may have to consider whether the pupil needs his information presented more immediately and less sequentially in the short or long term, or whether we need to keep all the structure the same, but reduce the amount of work.

Why is the child displaying this behaviour? 'I am displaying behaviour difficulties because …'	What can the teacher/TA do?
■ 'I'm being prevented from completing a strongly learnt routine which I now feel compulsive about doing.' ■ 'I've started this 'and must do it or finish it.'	Teacher/TA could … ■ Create a new routine.
■ 'I'm being asked to leave a situation I want to remain in.' ■ 'I'm so engaged with this I can't leave it.'	Teacher/TA could … ■ Consider whether the child needs to do this activity less frequently but for longer, or whether the child requires a graduated warning so as to disengage himself.
■ I am experiencing demand overload ■ 'I cannot do all this today' ■ 'I am not clear how much I'm meant to do.'	Teacher/TA could … ■ Maintain work then relax routine but reduce the amount of work. Set work out so the child can see what he has to do.
■ 'I am experiencing cumulative stress.' ■ 'I have just had enough of everything and am in a state of high anxiety.'	Teacher/TA could … ■ Plan times of relaxation for the child. Help the child to learn relaxation techniques, e.g. deep breathing, etc.
■ 'I am experiencing sensory overload.' ■ 'I am finding it hard to tolerate the sensory input from' or 'the sound/ sight, smell, taste, touch, temperature etc. of this upsets me.'	Teacher/TA could … ■ Consider a child's particular sensory difficulties when planning where he sits, and what he does.
■ 'I am in need of sensory input.' ■ 'I enjoy this form of sensory feedback.'	Teacher/TA could … ■ Give the child something to squeeze, hold, look at, etc., that provides sensory feedback without the child seeking it inappropriately.

	Teacher/TA could …
■ 'I am having problems with processing what is being said to me.' ■ 'I cannot understand everything you're saying to me and don't know what I'm being asked to do.'	■ Reduce language. Increase visual instructions. Repeat instructions in the same words.
■ 'I am having problems understanding changes.' ■ 'I don't recognize what I have to do now and have no visual memory of this situation to help me.'	■ Use visual means to explain a change, e.g. writing on a timetable, filing a symbol in a finished pocket and continuing to practise change, initially by making it positive and enjoyable, etc.
■ 'I am anxious or fearful.' ■ 'I am having difficulty predicting what may happen.'	■ Use a timetable, use visual cues.
■ 'I am unsure of the usual rules of social conduct.' ■ 'Everyone else seems to know what to do or say but I don't.'	■ Visual cues, social stories, power cards.
■ 'I am not aware of the effect of my actions on others.' ■ 'I did not know this would upset people.'	■ Use visual cues, social stories, power cards.
■ 'I am a perfectionist and very competitive.' ■ 'I like to get things right and not make mistakes, because if it goes wrong it's spoiled.'	■ Use a social story or a power card. Write about what to do when mistakes are made.

Sensory overload can also contribute to cumulative stress. Children on the autism spectrum may find it hard to regulate and filter visual or auditory information, as well as information from smell, taste, touch or movement. Carl, a boy with severe autism, was very hyperactive and wherever possible was always 'on the move'. On one occasion, he was taken into a quiet room to work. As he entered the room there was no light on and he sat down calmly. His usual fidgeting movements stopped. As soon as the light went on, he immediately began moving his legs, and hands and was focused on stereotypic behaviours. Whenever lighting was reduced and the room was a little darker, he was much calmer. This led to some set relaxation periods being put into his day where he could sit in a sensory area with low-key lighting to help him feel calm.

Simplifying our approach to solving behaviour difficulties

When children on the autism spectrum are displaying challenging behaviours it can be very easy to think in complicated ways about why it might be happening and what to do about the difficulty. This section aims to help teachers and TAs simplify the problem-solving process.

When we have a good understanding of autism and we can see a behaviour is situation-specific it is possible to analyse what the child is finding difficult about the situation. This can often help us to identify what to try and do about it. However, by asking ourselves the question 'In this situation, what do we want him to do?' we can simplify the problem-solving process further.

When we analyse *why* a child may be displaying challenging behaviour we are searching for the reason for his behaviour, and we hope to find in our analysis what we need to do about it. This can be a very helpful approach and enable us to see some detail that we may not have noticed before. Initially it is important to observe and record information about behaviour so that we can be factual about what is really happening.

Sometimes the discussion about why and what is happening can remain guesswork to a degree. When analysing the difficulty ceases to give insights and instead begins to confuse us further, it can be helpful to take another approach. First, if we understand that the problem the pupil is experiencing is real, results from frustration, misunderstanding, beliefs or perceptions caused by autism, rather than any deliberate negative act on his part, then in a broad sense we know *why* he is behaving as he does. Knowing that the problem is genuine for the child helps us to start our problem solving from a position of empathy. We can then either build on what we have analysed, or even start without that information, by using some guiding questions to enable us to find solutions.

Some useful questions to help us clarify what we need to do are:

■ What specifically do we want the child to do in this situation?

■ How might we set up the situation differently or 'teach' the child how to respond?

Asking 'What do we want the child to do?' involves us in clearly defining what we would usually expect someone to understand in a situation. It is important to state explicitly what might usually be implicit or hidden in terms of expected behaviour.

The second question involves us considering what we are going to do to support and enable the child to do the behaviour. This question also considers whether we need to manage the circumstances so that the child knows what to do or whether we need to help the child to get the right information so that he can do what is expected. The strategy we select needs to match the child's cognitive level so that the child learns to replace this behaviour at the right understanding level for him.

Below are examples of behaviour difficulties and how the use of these guiding questions can help us to consider what can be done to establish new, positive responses.

Example 1.
Difficulties with 'waiting'

Nathan becomes edgy and sometimes aggressive when he has to wait for a period of time. If we consider how autism is affecting him in this scenario we could assume that he may be:

- Unsure how long he will be in that situation.

- Unsure what 'waiting' actually means and what to do during the waiting time.

- Unsure what is to happen after this situation and so is edgy during it.

We may understand that any or all of these are causing him to exhibit difficult behaviour when he is put in a 'waiting' situation, or there may also be other factors.

If we are able to analyse and apply our knowledge of autism to the problem-solving process this may be helpful in understanding the child's genuine difficulty and in considering what we need to do to change his reaction.

Another way to simplify this process is to ask ourselves, 'What do we want him to *do* in this situation?' When the child has to, 'Wait' we really want the child *to sit and relax* for a period of time until circumstances change. Our range of 'waiting' strategies therefore needs to include things that the child finds relaxing to make the time he spends 'waiting' feel more definite and not stressful.

Depending on the pupil's interests, age and level of understanding, ideas might include the child having something to do which he finds relaxing and absorbing while he is waiting, e.g. a favourite book, a favourite magazine, a bag of toys or items he really loves, favourite music to listen to through headphones, etc.

How might we set up the situation differently or 'teach' the child how to respond? One approach we could consider is familiarizing him with what he needs to do by creating times in the day when he practises short waiting times which are not associated with those times which up to now he has found stressful. We can select times for him to look at or use his favourite activity and associate it with 'waiting', so that he immediately sees it as a positive experience.

When a pupil is happy with the physical arrangements, we could also consider how we ensure that the spoken, written or picture of the word 'wait' is not something for the pupil to be anxious about. When we have a comfortable activity that the child likes to do, the activity itself may become the cue for waiting.

Once the child is happier in the waiting situation or situations that were difficult for him, we can consider if we need to introduce the concept of waiting, so that we provide a longer-term solution to the problem. Depending on the child's age or level of understanding, this might be something to be done at that time, or may be something that the child is not yet ready for and may need to revisit later.

When teaching a child about why we may need to wait and what to do when we do, we need to consider how best to visually present the information. For example, if the child is a good reader and understands what he reads, you may want to write, 'Waiting for bus – sit and look at your book' on his timetable.

The child may need a sign, symbol, picture or photo to accompany his activity and learn that this is what 'wait' means in a number of contexts.

For a pupil who is able to generalize his understanding of waiting still further, other information about what waiting is about, in what kinds of situations it occurs and what the pupil can do when asked to wait in different contexts, could be presented either in a social story, or by using a power card strategy as described in Chapter 3.

Example 2.
Difficulty: switching lights on and off every time the child enters a room or leaves a room and sometimes during lessons

What do we want the child to do? We want him to ignore the light switches and concentrate on what he should be doing. For some children we therefore need to help them to ignore the light switches, for others we need to help them understand what they have to do, so that they can remain engaged with it.

One or more of the following suggestions may be useful in setting up circumstances differently to manage their behaviour or teach a new response:

- Covering the light switches so the child no longer sees them, which may prevent him from starting the behaviour.

- Providing the child with a clear reason to go into rooms and be clear about why he is going in a room so that he remains focused on this rather than on other details such as light switches.

- Presenting written/pictorial information which lets the child know what to do or not to do.

- Presenting written or pictoral information which lets the child know when and why we switch on lights and what lights are used for.

Example 3.
Difficulty: Jack talks on and on, and is not easy to interrupt or stop

Jack wants to talk a lot about his favourite subject, sharks, but will not accept that sometimes his peers or adults want to talk about other things.

What do we want Jack to do? We want Jack to enjoy some time talking about his interests but to accept talking about other subjects too and at other times not talking at all but concentrating on his work.

How might we set the circumstances up differently to enable this to happen or teach the child about when and where he can talk about his interests?

One or more of the following suggestions may be useful in setting the circumstances to manage this behaviour or teach a new response:

- Provide times in the day for him to talk about his interests and show when these are on his timetable.

- Use a written list of what is to be talked about, cross or tick them off to indicate they have been talked about (Figure 13).

TALKING INSECTS CARD

Spiders (2 types) ☐

Bees (1 type) ☐

Ants (2 types) ☐

Figure 13 A talk card with a written list of what is to be talked about

When using a 'talking card' list ensure that the information on the card is recorded differently in terms of how much is being talked about and in what order so that we help the child to be flexible.

- Use a social story about what friends like to talk about.

- Make a set of relevant social question cards and play games asking these to provide sources of other conversation starters or topics.

- Provide clear information about when the child needs to be quiet and working and when talk time is possible.

Ideas for teaching new skills in a clear and structured way really can help to replace behaviours which are preventing learning.

The Case Study exercise on pages 101–2 offers a problem-solving scenario. The exercise can be used by teachers and TAs to review how using simple questions can help staff work out what to do.

TRY THIS!

If a child wants to talk on and on about his favourite special interest try using a 'let's talk' folder. The folder should have an area for individual pictures related to the subject on the left and a finish pocket on the right. The child can be taught that when 'time to talk' is written on the timetable he may have short sessions using this folder. Teach the child that when the person listening has heard enough the picture will be filed in the finish pocket so that a clear signal is given for the child to move on to the next picture to be talked about. Maintain interest by using a variety of pictures and maintain flexibility by always presenting the folder with different amounts of pictures to talk about each time. This will ensure that the 'let's talk time' is realistically possible within the school day.

Motivation or relaxation and its impact on behaviour

For most teachers, teaching assistants and pupils the use of reinforcing activities, or things, is a common classroom tool. Often the reward system or rewards themselves are used to ensure that pupils are given incentives or motivators to work hard. This system is often used with children who are on the autism spectrum and can be very successful, as with other children. Sometimes, however, pupils on the autism spectrum may work effectively and may seem to understand the reward system fully when in fact what they understand is the routine of work and then reward. This does not mean that this system is not a good one, as it may be one of the structures that the child feels secure working within, but it is important to recognize that the reason why it is working may not always be exactly the same as why it works for other pupils who are not on the spectrum.

Alternatively some pupils on the autism spectrum really do not see their special interests as rewards but rather see them as 'relaxers'. These pupils may well work more effectively if they are allowed time to do their relaxer prior to work rather than following it. That way they are calm and able to respond in the work situation because they have had the space and time to relax in readiness for learning.

Establishing a work-then-reward ethic is quite a natural one for teachers and teaching assistants to use, whereas establishing a relax-then-work ethic may not be such a usual approach and may require us to make a shift in our thinking and planning to accommodate it as a different approach. Changing our approach like this is necessary only when working the other way round does not seem to be eliciting the best work or the best behaviour from pupils who are on the autism spectrum. When faced with this situation it always seems worth trying to change things round.

The exercise on pages 101–2 allows teachers and TAs to practise application of the key questions for working out behaviour difficulties with a range of difficulties which they may encounter in different school contexts or the questions could be applied to a particular behaviour difficulty which staff want to investigate.

QUESTIONS FOR WORKING IT OUT

A CASE STUDY EXERCISE

Consider the following questions and how they help to clarify ways forward in resolving behaviour challenges with the example given below. Then apply all this to any of the other examples of behaviour challenges presented in the next section.

What does the child do now?

Brian tears up his work and gets angry when he makes a mistake.

What might the child not understand or know to do in this situation because of his autism?

Brian may not know how to put the mistake right. He may feel he has to start all over again. He may not be able to listen and process what he could do. He may not be able to accept guidance from those around him.

What specifically do we want the child to do in this situation?

For Brian to remain calm, select from a guided choice about what he can do in this situation so that he can continue his work.

How do we teach the child what we want him to do?

First, teaching Brian to remain calm, rather than go immediately to an angry response, could be an important first step. This might involve teaching Brian to breathe in and out several times, first in calm situations and then in all situations involving stress, or teaching him to look at a favourite subject picture with a guidance message on it. For example, if cars are a favourite subject it could be a car picture with a relevant relaxation slogan on it.

Second, what approach or approaches could work in teaching Brian to overcome the difficulty? At this stage all ideas are welcome and can go down as potential strategies to select from.

- Make a change of writing implement such as a pen with an eraser.
- Use a wipe-off board as a spelling practice board before he puts his work on paper.
- Let Brian watch someone else making a mistake and be asked to help the other person decide what to do. (Record Brian's ideas on what to do as a set of guidelines to be used in the future.)
- Write a list of class rules which include one that says mistakes are allowed and suggest how they could be used to help us learn.

Write an explanation of how making mistakes can help us learn and how they can be put right. (Use the web or look up books which use social story formats, power card formats or other good written material for ideas.)

QUESTIONS FOR WORKING IT OUT

- What does the child do now?

- What may the child not understand or know to do in this situation?

- What specifically do we want the child to do in this situation?

- How do we teach the child what we want him to do in this situation?

Some behaviours to think about

- When it is David's turn on the computer, he will not leave when it is time for him to finish.

- Sarah takes food off the plates of others.

- Shane does not line up when the other children do, even though he is told on a daily basis.

- Rachel tells tales on other children and then gets very angry when told not to.

- Martin attacks other children if they cry.

- Tony grabs toys from other children.

- Ian works well and then, on the last bit, he just gets really cross and spoils it.

Working together to solve behaviour challenges

It is important for teachers and teaching assistants to work together to find the most effective solution to challenging behaviour. Behaviour difficulties can have an impact on the morale and self esteem of teachers and TAs.

> Whenever I worked with this child he played up, and with the other TA he was pretty good. People said not to take it personally, but how can you not when he was better with other people than with me?
>
> (Teaching assistant)

When working with children on the autism spectrum it can be important to gather information about the pupil as well as about the particular behaviour challenge he is displaying. A SWOT form is used on page 104 as a starting point for gathering information or considering what information we already have.

SWOT tools were originally used in business for assessing strengths, weaknesses, opportunities and threats. The form has been adapted and has qualifying questions to help focus our thinking on information which surrounds the behaviour challenge a pupil is displaying and may give us clues as to how we can combine information to form effective strategies.

The overall goal of the form is to help us consider:

- How can we use each strength.

- How we can reduce the weaknesses.

- How we can make the most of each opportunity.

- How we can minimize factors that might undermine our action.

Using SPACE for solving challenging behaviour

When Sencos, senior teachers or any staff members are trying to support colleagues facing complex behaviour, it is important to acknowledge the reality for the staff involved, along with the belief that by taking some simple steps to decrease stress for both staff and pupils an appropriate strategy will emerge. When under stress, the empathy of colleagues can sometimes be seen, at best, as interfering and, at worst, as 'superior'. Sencos, department heads, senior teachers or whoever is providing support for colleagues faced with a child on the autism spectrum who is exhibiting behaviour difficulties, needs to consider the way in which they can provide effective support for any colleague who need it. It is important to provide time for staff to talk about the difficulties being encountered and time to listen to what is being felt and experienced by staff before any ways of interpreting the behaviour or strategy suggestions are considered. Often colleagues wanting to help others offer immediate ideas for ways to solve the problem which may be relevant but which are better considered later when staff are ready to hear and evaluate them. Equally, teachers and TAs have to be willing to seek or receive support and guidance and see it as part of taking positive action.

SWOT : A TOOL FOR TEAMWORK AND POSITIVE BEHAVIOUR PLANNING

STRENGTHS

What good personal qualities does the child have?

What skills does the child have?

What special interests or motivators does the child have?

WEAKNESSES

What behaviour challenge does the child present?

When and where does he/she do it?

Why do we think he/she is doing this behaviour? How will we find out whether this is the right view?

OPPORTUNITIES

When does the child behave well? What does this tell us?

Who can give us more information or support in relation to this child and his/her behaviour, e.g. parents, other staff, etc.?

THREATS

What strategies have we tried? How did they work? What may have undermined them and caused them not to work?

Where and why might we find it hard to carry out any strategy we decide upon?

Helping Children with Autistic Spectrum Disorders to Learn, Paul Chapman Publishing © Mary Pittman 2007

When providing support to colleagues or considering our own support needs, it can be important to:

- Allow sufficient time for staff to talk, and tell their 'story' of the difficulty and the impact it is having on them, the child and the other pupils.

- Reframe the child's difficulties for the staff by explaining where and how autism is causing the behaviour and as a consequence help staff to depersonalize the situation.

- Identify all the positive aspects of working with the pupil, his strengths, interests, etc. Consider where and when the pupil is calm, relaxed and working well.

- Establish a *temporary plan* to break the cycle of stress and enable the child to feel generally happier and more relaxed in school. This plan may mean that demands are lowered or avoided. It is important to remember that this plan is temporary and its goal is to prevent or reduce challenging behaviour. Stopping the child being in a situation which he reacts badly to can prevent accumulative stress and a routine response becoming established.

- Create opportunities for the teachers and/or TAs to be active in seeking information as part of their problem-solving. It is important that the staff directly involved seek the information and feel empowered in the problem solving process. Sources of information may include the child himself, parents, other professionals in the school, Communication and Interaction teams, etc.

- Initially, keep specific behaviour meetings short but regular. Focus, initially, on understanding the stress levels of the pupil and the staff, establishing a temporary plan and seeking additional support and information. Once the plan is in place and is having a positive impact, meetings can then focus on what action to take in the longer term.

- Ensure staff are aware of the school's behaviour policy and interventions and help them with the necessary paperwork where needed.

When children on the autism spectrum are stressed, staff may need to think about creating times for the child to have 'space' from the situations they are finding difficult.

The acronym SPACE can help to provide a useful framework for the problem-solving process when supporting children on the autism spectrum displaying challenging behaviour. The points above should be applied using the SPACE sheet on page 106.

Once the level of stress and consequent difficult behaviour have reduced then a plan of how to teach new skills can be addressed. Schools who encourage staff to share information and act as soon as they see that a pupil on the autism spectrum is experiencing difficulty are likely to help both the staff and the student, as it will ensure that a behaviour or negative routine will not have much time to become established.

USING THE SPACE APPROACH TO PREVENTING AND PROBLEM-SOLVING BEHAVIOUR DIFFICULTIES

Stress

	Initial judgement										Follow-up	Follow-up	Follow-up
Pupil	1	2	3	4	5	6	7	8	9	10			
Staff	1	2	3	4	5	6	7	8	9	10			

Prevention

Temporary plan to reduce stress, or prevent further escalation of the behaviour. Consider whether you are applying this plan to a child displaying situation-specific behaviour challenges or to a child who is displaying random incidents of behaviour challenges.

Action

What will we do longer-term to problem solve? What longer-term strategies and resources could help?

Calming environments or extras

What does this child enjoy and feel calm doing that we can use as positives to motivate, relax and enable him to cope and be successful?

Suggestions for helping children with autism to learn

PIECES OF THE BEHAVIOUR PROBLEM-SOLVING PUZZLE

- Understand behaviour as a form of communication from a child with autism.

- Recognize the difference between situation-specific behaviour and regular but unpredictable behaviour.

- Ask the question 'In this situation what do we want the child to do?'

- Create new behaviour routines for a child with autism and teach what is appropriate to do or say.

- Work together using strengths/weaknesses/opportunities/threats information to support teamwork planning.

- Use SPACE approach as a framework for managing challenging behaviour.

FURTHER READING

- Dunn Buron, K. and Curis, M. (2003) *The Incredible Five-point Scale. Assisting Students with Autism Spectrum Disorders in Understanding Social Interactions and Controlling their Emotional Responses.* Shawnee Mission KS: Autism Asperger Publishing.

- Smith Myles, B., Trautman, M. L. and Schelvan, R.L. (2004) *The Hidden Curriculum. Practical Solutions for Understanding Unstated Rules in Social Situations.* Shawnee Mission KS: Autism Asperger Publishing.

- Whitaker, P. (2001) *Challenging Behaviour and Autism. Making Sense – Making progress. A Guide to Preventing and Managing Challenging Behaviour for Parents and Teachers.* London: National Autistic Society.

Frequently Asked Questions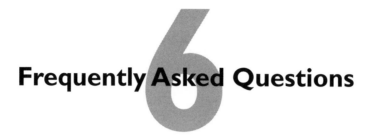

This chapter considers examples of questions frequently asked by teachers and TAs working with children on the autism spectrum. The replies given to questions cannot provide a successful outcome for every child, in every situation, and are not provided as definitive answers. However, the replies provided are suggestions for teachers and TAs to try. They are based on approaches that have been used by teachers and which provide some principles of good practice which could be applied when working with other children. The replies aim to share experiences and encourage further reflection on the questions being asked.

The questions used in this chapter are a selection of the many that teachers and teaching assistants have asked. The chapter is divided into sections which cover:

- General questions.

- Specific questions relating to teaching children with autism and severe learning difficulties.

- Specific questions relating to teaching children with autism in the early years.

- Specific questions relating to teaching children in primary schools.

- Specific questions relating to teaching children in secondary schools.

Although the questions are divided in this way, it is worth considering some of the questions and replies in areas which do not directly relate to the age or developmental level of pupils that you work with, as they may contain useful information or clarify principles that can be further adapted to your own setting.

General questions

The aim of this section is to provide some examples which cross age and developmental ranges.

Can a visual approach really help a child in developing a work ethic?

Some pupils on the autism spectrum need a more visual system for providing them with information about what comes next or what they have to look forward to when work is finished. As with all visual strategies these need to be presented at the appropriate level for them to access this information. This can be considered a 'work then reward' system but I have often found that it is more effective to consider it a 'work then relax' system, as the child may want to know when the pressure is off him for a while. Using this description can help us to remember that what we are asking the child to do is learn this work ethic and that it can be difficult for him to learn. The child may not be equating his time doing something he enjoys as reward because he has done the previous work. Instead he can be doing the 'work' activity as a step in getting towards his more favoured one. Another consideration is that he is keen to do the work set for him so he can obtain time doing an activity that he likes because when doing it he feels calm and not under stress. The importance of the relaxing or rewarding activity being presented visually is that it can be seen by the child and used by the teacher to remind the child rather than reminding through the use of too much language, which might be confusing. This visual tool, like a number of others, allows the child to have a reminder which enables him to remain independent of an adult, and significantly it is a visual promise which builds trust.

The following points may help to answer this question further and relate to points made in Chapter 4. Some younger children or those pupils with substantial developmental learning difficulties can require 'work then relax' systems to be shown to a child visually on 'First and Then' or 'Now and Next' boards. These can be presented using objects, icons or symbols, or by written words.

Other pupils may need rewarding activities positioned on their timetable and may need decisions to be made and shown to them on the timetable as to where in the day these reward times are permitted. For some pupils this also helps in ensuring that they can leave their favoured rewarding activities and come back to working more easily because they can see when they can continue later in the day or have another session of this reward.

Some children may respond to the 'work then reward' system but initially may need more time doing the reward activity and less on the work activity. Once the routine of this system is in place the time spent and the demands of the work activity can be increased. Some pupils on the autism spectrum need to know what they are working for. They may need a visual reminder of what they are aiming for. Where rewards are to be given in token form and saved towards a specific reward. There are many inventive ways that teachers and TAs find to present these visual reward/relax systems, e.g. using a picture of the reward or a picture of the reward cut into sections and compiled a piece at a time is one of the many ways that can be used.

Certain pupils on the autism spectrum do not understand or feel motivated by working for something, even if they do like the idea of that activity or reward. With pupils who are very stressed or who do not respond to this approach, it can be worth considering defining a 'relax then work' approach. There are some children and adults on the autism spectrum who respond well to a period of doing an activity they enjoy as a means of reducing stress, which in turn means they are able to focus on the work they are then asked to do. This approach still achieves the aim of establishing a work ethic: it just does so from a different start point.

Are visual supports always necessary?

Sometimes pupils are functioning well in a situation without a specialist strategy of any kind and if this is the case intervening and using a visual strategy may not be necessary.

Some children, however, need a step-by-step plan of visual supports to enable them to develop independence in specific routines rather than relying on verbal direction.

Other children may not need visual supports for most situations but may suddenly find themselves stressed by a new or unexpected situation. In these situations a simple drawing or writing down the key concept or instruction as an alternative to giving spoken instructions or information can enable the student to follow what is needed without anxiety.

There are also times when children or students have become so stressed that visual structures and visual prompts have started to become demands in themselves and are therefore no longer a support. On these occasions it is important to look at the level at which the visual support is presented and the way in which the visual support is being used to ensure that both are easy and relaxing for the child. It may be helpful to introduce a new system at the right level for these children, or observe to see if any element of the existing approach is not clear and could be changed to be more effective. An example of this would be a student, who could easily read a timetable or schedule but did not want to mark off when each part was completed. He sometimes become lost because of not doing so. In observing him it was clear that he enjoyed any opportunity to fold paper over, and this was a strength. His subsequent timetable was made so that each step could be folded over when completed. This ensured it remained a tool that was significant in his life, because he enjoyed using it.

Why do visual supports sometimes not work?

There are all sorts of reasons why visual learning supports of different types and levels work or do not work. Some of the questions worth asking ourselves when using a visual tool to help a child learn or change a behaviour could be;

- Are we addressing the specific information the child needs?

- Are we sure our visual cues are at the right level? Are they visual enough?

- Are we familiarizing the child with what the visual tool does and teaching its use and meaning clearly enough?

- Are we talking too much as we use them?

One reason why a visual support, like a timetable, does not work is that an already stressed child has began to see the timetable as a stress in itself, rather than a helpful system for giving him information. For example, a visual timetable used to cue the child to the next lesson or activity may feel to the child that a demand is being made upon him. In these situations staff can feel disempowered, as something which they viewed as a necessary tool has let them down. However, the child may feel stressed by his visual timetable because an adult is speaking to him about his timetable rather than letting him use his timetable independently. If we are verbally cueing a child to the timetable, and naming the activities and using the visual timetable to back up our spoken directions instead of replacing them, then a child can really feel that he is having to process language, something he finds difficult, as well as use a timetable. A first step to test this out would be to stop talking as the child looks at his timetable or is given his timetable cue. Setting up the timetable so that the whole process of coming to it and using it is as independent as possible and reliant on good visuals rather than verbal cues is important in ensuring it is useful, comfortable and desirable for the child to use.

I don't know where independent work sessions can fit into the school day.

If the goal of our education programme for a child is independence, then every lesson, every routine and every situation the child is in needs to ensure that we are maximizing his or her independence in taking part. This question, however, relates directly to times of using an independent work/study system at a table in the classroom whereby existing skills are being practised and the reply given focuses on this.

The timing of independent work/study sessions needs to fit into the structure that suits both the class timetable and the individual pupil's needs. It often becomes obvious as to where in the day other lessons or activities are difficult and where a child or student would benefit from taking time to work alone.

- Sometimes independent work/study sessions can become a regular part of the Literacy or Numeracy Hour for a pupil.

- Sometimes independent work/study sessions can be for regular short periods during the day for an individual pupil. For some children these sessions are more useful than free choice times as they provide a calm low stress time.

- Sometimes independent work/study sessions can be used to help a pupil who can concentrate only for part of a lesson. The student then needs to remain calm and be able to continue quietly working alone without the continued pressures of concentrating on language-based teaching.

- With some children who have autism and severe learning difficulties, having a short session of independent work on their timetable each time they enter the classroom (e.g. start of school day, after break, after lunch, etc.) can be useful. It helps them to settle into the classroom and become ready to receive information about other activities on their schedule once a calm working atmosphere has been established.

How can special interests be managed effectively?

Children on the autism spectrum often have special interests, which can be useful to use as motivating or relaxing activities, and may give teachers and TAs useful areas that can be used in establishing a balance of work and relaxation/enjoyment.

Teachers and TAs do need to help pupils in managing their special interests so that they remain a positive motivating force or a way of relaxing and preparing to focus. However, occasionally a special interest becomes so engaging for a child that it is hard for him to disengage and leave the activity.

If a child can engage in his chosen special interest, then disengage as appropriate and return to directed learning, the special interest is really useful and can be very supportive to the child's learning.

Some pupils on the autism spectrum need to know and see visually on a written or picture timetable when they will be having time with their special interests. They also need to know that there are a number of opportunities for them to do their favourite activity in the day and also when this will happen. For some pupils, this helps them to leave their special interest when asked, as they can be shown on the timetable that there are other occasions when they can return to it.

With some children their special interest needs considerable time to set up and carry out. When they are not given enough time to engage and disengage, the teacher may feel that the special interest has a negative aspect rather than being a motivating, relaxing or supportive strategy to use. In these circumstances, time doing the special interest activity has to be planned in carefully.

Are all pupils on the autism spectrum visual learners?

Although most young people on the autism spectrum do tend to learn more effectively from what they see or read, there are some who appear to be strong auditory or kinaesthetic learners and require a mixture of learning styles.

However, presenting information to the student is usually most effective when presented visually. For some children it is important to see and hear what is expected, for others to see what is expected of them by doing it, and for others to recognize that other sensory cues are accompanying what we see happening. An example of this would be when a child in an early years class, or a developmentally young child, is given an object that depicts circle time and a piece of music is also played to indicate that we are now starting group time.

Do children on the autism spectrum deliberately misbehave or are their behaviour difficulties the result of their autism?

Teachers and TAs often wonder if some of the behaviours that children on the autism spectrum are displaying are deliberately orchestrated or used to manipulate situations.

Usually children on the autism spectrum are behaving in a reactive way to situations that occur and their responses appear to be the result of their difficulties in thinking flexibly and their misunderstanding of social situations. Sometimes children want routines and situations to be done as they have visualized them, and this can look controlling and deliberate. However, it is often more about establishing sameness.

For most children the confusion that autism causes is the sole cause of behaviour difficulties. For example, their difficulties with engagement and disengagement can mean that children appear as if they are not willing to listen or do what is being asked when in fact at that moment they may not be able to hear or attend to what is being requested of them. The difficulties a child has with understanding the social factors which rely on us 'reading between the lines' and picking up on subtle cues as well as all the other areas of difficulty that children on the spectrum encounter means that they are likely to feel frustrated in understanding what we want from them and why we want it.

Some children do learn that their behaviour can bring about a reaction in others which they may notice and seem to enjoy. Some children will want to repeat the routine that brings about this chain of events, while others may enjoy the reaction they obtain. But this tends to be more about the fascination it may hold for them than any understanding of the effect they are having on someone else. In the nature of things, being on the autism spectrum means that an understanding of how others feel and think is unlikely to be a consideration in how they behave.

Some students who are high functioning or have Asperger's syndrome, however, may behave according to strong beliefs that they hold about justice or fairness. Some students act on their beliefs and see such behaviour as justifiable.

Why do children sometimes go back to negative behaviours that they seemed to have stopped?

Sometimes children start to use behaviours that they have not used for some time. This can feel disappointing to staff or parents and could be for a number of reasons. One reason seems to be that the child recalls behaviours that he did last time he was feeling stressed or confused in a situation. Sometimes a child uses past behaviours as a response to a set of circumstances his visual memory recalls. Some children on the spectrum only have a small range of responses that they can draw on to communicate that they are feeling worried, unclear of what to do, etc. and do not have the words to say what they feel and so their behaviours are their only way to communicate what they are finding hard.

Sometimes children have just forgotten what to do, or need visually reminding of what to do, so that they can behave appropriately. Others cannot generalize the behaviour they had learnt to do in one situation and do not realize that the same behaviour is required in this context until it is taught to them.

Specific questions: autism and severe learning difficulties

Why might a non-speaking child with autism and severe learning difficulties try to alter their visual timetable by rearranging the pictures or removing them?

There are several possible scenarios which might make a child behave in this way. Sometimes a child with dual difficulties is unsure about the differences between their timetable/schedule and their communication board. Therefore sometimes a child will use his timetable to request certain activities that he enjoys. The child is therefore using the timetable to make requests as if it is a communication board. It is important to ensure that a child has a communication board to use for such expressions and that he is referred to it. Then, if appropriate, as part of the answer to his request he can be shown on his timetable when he will be having that activity.

Occasionally a child with dual difficulties of this complexity and severity sees that his own timetable is different from the order presented on a peer's timetable. Sometimes he will change the order on his own timetable to be the same as a peer's. The child who does this is creating sameness by 'matching' rather than understanding or following his timetable as a source of information for himself. This child does not have ownership of his timetable and may need his timetable to be changed in some way to make it more meaningful. It would be useful to reassess what the child understands from his timetable by observing whether he goes independently to places and whether he follows his system independently. If he does not, his actions may be showing that the timetable is just a routine to him and not at the right level to be really useful in helping him be independent.

Why might a child with autism and severe learning difficulties want to work at high speed through each activity on the timetable?

Sometimes children on the autism spectrum do not understand the time frames in which they are being asked to do things and may consider that something you are talking about or showing them that is for later in the day is really for now. Some children feel that they just need to work through a set of activities to have them removed from the timetable, and see their timetable as a list of things to be worked through and completed as quickly as possible rather than a system for ordering their day.

This tends to imply that they are not ready for a sequence of activities yet. The child may also need more clarity in terms of the work system for each activity and clues as to how long each activity may be and what clearly depicts that it is finished. Try giving the child his timetable information more immediately or on a first/then basis rather than a long sequence.

'I am working with pupils who have autism and severe learning difficulties and I am having problems varying the content of independent work for each pupil. What can I do?'

As children with dual difficulties, autism and SLD, for example, are more reliant on adults managing their work content and systems than some other pupils there is a need to consider a number of options when individualizing independent work systems for pupils with this level of complex needs.

The following reply considers just some of the numerous range of individual difficulties a child may demonstrate when considering the content of independent work tasks. One very important factor to consider is: do we have a repertoire of activities that this child can successfully do independently even when he is stressed or not well? Some children vary in their performance owing to a number of factors and so it is always important to have a set of activities that the child can do in any circumstances and find them calming and reassuring.

When changing or varying independent work activities some pupils need one or two activities which they are familiar with left in their work tray or basket so that they feel comfortable that they can achieve the set tasks and then they are happy to do other activities which are new.

Some pupils, however, need the whole set of activities in their work tray or basket to be changed, because if they recognize them they visually recall the order of the tasks they did previously and expect it to be the same.

Some pupils benefit from always doing independent work at their own workstation or work table whenever they enter their classroom e.g. first thing on arrival in school, whenever break time or lunchtime is over, for example. This sometimes provides a stable period of work at a key transition time when they may be unsure about what may be expected of them when they enter the classroom.

If work trays or baskets are used to provide this calm level of transition throughout a school day there needs to be enough work trays, e.g. four per day. Work trays may not take very long for pupils to do, e.g. from a few minutes to fifteen minutes. It is important to make judgements about how many activities should be in each work tray and how long you want each work session to last as well as considering what is supportive and possible for each individual pupil.

During independent work sessions it is important that a teacher or teaching assistant uses this time to observe how tasks are being achieved, the number of tasks, whether any specific IEP targets in relation to independent work are being met. It is important not to actively teach the pupil during these sessions. If the child needs any support to learn an aspect of becoming more independent in the process of doing independent work then back prompting in silence is likely to be the most effective means. It prevents the pupil becoming prompt-dependent on language or physical actions that are more overt.

What is the most effective way to teach the use of an independent work system?

As far as using an independent work system is concerned, the only area that should require teaching is the actual procedure for getting work, doing it, and placing it somewhere when it is finished. The content of tasks and activities should require no teaching, as they should be activities that a child can do with ease and with no intervention by an adult. If an activity is not done successfully without intervention from an adult it should be removed from independent work and taught, in one-to-one sessions possibly, but only put back into independent work once the child can do it with ease and without support. If an adult intervenes in independent work whilst it is in progress this will immediately interrupt the flow and can break down the system, creating a situation in which the child expects help and may even become prompt-dependent.

A child does often need teaching to:

■ Pick up a task from a work tray/work basket, etc.

■ Open the pack, if it is in one, and do it.

■ Place the finished task in the finished tray or basket.

■ Do the next activity in the work tray/basket.

Once the child is set up with the 'work to do' tray on his left, the 'finished' tray on his right and sufficient space in front of him to do the task the adult needs to observe if the child will pull across or pick up the first activity on his left and do it. The adult should intervene only if the child does not begin his independent work and follow the process. The teacher or TA observing needs to intervene only where necessary and should do so without speaking and by using a physical back-prompt. The back-prompt can be very important, as it means that the adult is using the child's own movements rather than causing a distraction or prompt dependence. Any action such as pointing and directing a child as to what to do or speaking instructions can easily become something which the child waits for. This prevents the whole aim of independent working.

Specific questions: early years

What if a young child with ASD does not like following a timetable and directing him or her to go to their timetable triggers a behaviour problem?

Sometimes children have begun to feel negative about a timetable because it gives stress rather than alleviates it. This implies that the child is finding the predictive mode of the timetable difficult or the communication of the timetable event stressful. If this is so, the teacher needs to think about transitioning to the schedule.

This can be because the timetable is not wholly visual but involves verbal instruction from us to go to the timetable, etc. In these situations teachers could try to direct a young child to his timetable by giving the child a card which he learns means go to the timetable rather than verbally directing him. This sometimes allows the child to be directed without using the verbal direction which has developed negative connotations.

Other children can become so stressed that each time they are cued to an activity using a timetable they feel they are encountering a demand which they cannot cope with. Try putting on the timetable, or directing the child to activities he enjoys first so he feels comfortable with using a timetable or cues.

What can you do when a young child does not want to do what is on the timetable because he has no desire to work?

It is important that a child sees the timetable as useful and as something to enjoy and that it reduces stress rather than causes it. When first starting out to teach a young child to use a timetable it can be good to develop its use step by step rather than expecting the child to just automatically gain from its use.

Where the child has a number of activities he or she likes these can be arranged on the timetable so that the child is happy to let the timetable direct him to the activities in the order they appear on the timetable. The child is here learning to accept direction and the ordering of activities. Then other activities which the adult wishes to put into the timetable can be added gradually and for very short periods until the child is happy to have the activity incorporated into his schedule.

What ways can young children on the autism spectrum be encouraged to play?

There are a number of ways that children on the autism spectrum can be taught and supported in play. There are children who really benefit from being given the opportunity to lead play actions by the adult copying what the child does. Some approaches such as the Son Rise programme uses this way of encouraging interaction and play. Other children benefit from the play area and the toys they use being structured so that they are clear how to use them.

Questions: primary school issues

I have set up an independent work system for a pupil but he is getting some of the questions on the worksheet wrong and needs help with them. What should I do?

As the whole aim of any independent work system is for the pupil to do the work totally himself it is important not to step in and correct any work that the pupil does incorrectly. It is better in this context to allow the work to be left as the child has done it and to allow the pupil to finish the work independently even if at this stage it is not correct. The fact that this piece of work was not able to be done provides us with insight into what we need to place as tasks for independent work. Independent work does mean that we try to ensure the child does it alone but it also requires us to be constantly assessing where it is going well and where the child is not succeeding so that we can make small adjustments where necessary. If the child is getting work incorrect remove any activities that a pupil cannot achieve independently so that the goal of independent work/study is maintained. Any work or skills that the child is having difficulty with should instead be taught in one-to-one teaching sessions.

How can a calendar be made more visual in terms of the current day?

Some pupils need to have an overview of the week. This can be particularly the case at home. The child needs to know which days he is at home and which days he is at school or where a child sees one parent at alternate weekends. Whatever the purpose the weekly calendar, where it is needed, may not be obvious to a child in terms of recognizing the current day during the week. One way of highlighting the current day is to attach an outline strip of coloured card over the current day which can slide along to each day as the week progresses and draws the child's attention to the current day but allows them to also see the other days of the week.

What arrangements need to be made to help children cope with break times and use of the playground?

Some pupils on the autism spectrum find playtimes difficult because they are often less structured than lesson time and they have to rely upon social language and social under-standing, both of which pose difficulties for these students. If written or picture systems are proving useful in class time then these give us a clue as to the kinds of systems that the child may require during break or lunchtime. Work systems for break-time activities can be as useful as for class activities.

Some pupils need to follow a playtime schedule or timetable so that they have direction over the playtime period. Some pupils need to look at a playtime activity choice board to help them decide what to do. Other pupils need either social stories or visual reminders about what to say or do in playtime situations.

Some pupils find that they do not cope well with indoor play when outside playtimes are cancelled due to weather. Often we call this 'wet play' although this language is not always the most helpful for a child on the autism spectrum. Therefore agree the words which describe the situation best, e.g. classroom playtime or inside play/outside play, etc.

Making an activities choice board so that a pupil can choose what they do over the inside playtime can be helpful, as can ensuring that where possible activities are spread out and in defined places. Teaching a child how the weather affects playtimes is very important in the long term.

Questions: secondary school issues

What kinds of timetables can be used in secondary contexts with students so that they are age-appropriate?

Timetables for secondary-age students, as for other students, need to match a student's needs in terms of their developmental understanding, interests and a mode that the indi-vidual student feels he/she will use. Some students need their timetable to be presented in ways that might otherwise be used in a primary setting.

Some secondary schools use the same timetable as used for other students and find that no changes are needed, as the student can follow the format easily. Other secondary schools find that using a highlighter pen, or enlarging or rearranging the information, is helpful. Some schools use Filofax-style calendars, a daily diary, notebooks or electronic palmtops.

What kinds of strategies are useful to pupils in preparation for the transition from Year 6 in primary school to starting Year 7 in secondary school?

Most primary and secondary schools are now aware of the need for carefully planned transition arrangements for pupils on the autism spectrum and for other pupils with SEN. Strategies which are being found useful are transition visits, photographs of the staff or classroom areas, clear maps and opportunities to practise routes around the school, opportunities to practise reading timetables.

Some young people who are in Special School environments but are moving from primary school departments to secondary school departments may also require transition arrangements along similar lines.

Some pupils benefit from using social stories about their new school context, which can be introduced at the end of term and given to parents to use during the holidays as a tool for easing anxieties during the school holidays and to use on the first day as a guide for who they will meet and what will be expected.

How can pupils be helped to cope when the expected teacher for a lesson is away and there is a supply teacher?

Some students find it difficult to accept that their expected teacher is not taking the class when they arrive at the classroom.

Some students need to have a rule in place whereby if the usual teacher is not available the student can, on seeing this, make their way to their learning resource base and not enter the lesson. They can get on with work in that learning resource base for the duration of the lesson.

Some students can accept a verbal or written warning during the day about a lesson or staff change.

Some students can accept a teacher change because they have a consistent relationship with a TA. If a TA is away for any reason then information about what to do and where to go may need to be established in the same ways.

How can we help children to understand when there are changes of staff, for example when there are going to be different teaching assistants supporting a student?

At the end of a school year TA staff are sometimes asked to change roles and responsibilities. This can mean considerable difficulties for some students on the autism spectrum. Also there can be situations where a TA is moving away from his/her job. There needs to be a planned strategy so that a student on the autism spectrum can cope with these situations.

For most students who are at secondary level, and are able to follow written information easily, the most important thing is to ensure they have the factual information they need to be able to prepare and accept changes in their school day. Sometimes it is the reading of information that can be most helpful to a pupil. The creation of a written information sheet can be used to ensure that a student is given a warning about what to expect in terms of:

- Dates when things are occurring differently.

- The reasons why things are occurring differently.

- What will be happening instead of the usual arrangement.

- Which staff member they will be with for which lessons.

An example might be a student who had two TAs working with him for different parts of the school day and week. A circumstance arose whereby both the TAs were leaving within a few weeks of each other and before the end of the summer term. In this situation an information sheet was written out for the pupil which explained:

- The date when the first TA was leaving and where she was going to work in the future.

- The name of the TA covering those lessons (a known member of staff).

- The date when the second TA was leaving and where he was going.

- The name of the TA who was to cover these lessons, along with a photo, because this person was not known to the student.

The information sheet was read out to the student to explain the changes and the sheet was given to him to carry around and read as and when he needed to. A copy was also given to his parents and whenever he was unsure about any of the issues the sheet was used by the parents or TAs, Senco, etc., to ensure that the student understood and could cope with changes. A short meeting time was arranged for the student to meet new staff.

Why do some students have real problems with creative writing and what can be done about it?

When children are young one of the differences we often observe is how a child plays and in particular how a child plays imaginatively. In older years this difference can manifest itself further when students on the autism spectrum are expected to produce creative writing. In these situations students may need supportive frameworks to enable them to write sentences and paragraphs, and guidance as to what constitutes sentences for the beginning, middle and ending of their work. Students may require recording formats or maps for establishing their thoughts and ideas. Some students need to have clear explanations about the differences between fiction and non-fiction and ways of combining ideas from what they have seen so they create a new idea.

What do you do if a student is asking about and wanting to know why he/she is different from his/her peers?

It is important to consider carefully if, and when, a student is ready to consider his/her own differences and develop their own self-awareness of autism or Asperger's syndrome.

This decision needs to be discussed and planned between parents and school staff, and with outside agents who can guide the process, e.g. psychologists, outreach teachers from Communication and Interaction teams, etc. Before embarking on this work it is also very important to review relevant resources that can guide the process and use the principles of good practice that have emerged from staff who have been involved in this work.

One factor that is very important in this decision is whether the student has a good understanding of fact and fantasy, and can distinguish and balance information that is real with that which is not.

It is also helpful to ensure that the student views the autism or Asperger's syndrome as part of his/her life and importantly that they are an individual with the same likes, dislikes, opinions and responsibilities towards others as other individuals

This area should be approached carefully, with the full consent of parents and the involvement of all relevant professionals. The work should be planned so as to address the issue within a sound framework. The student needs to develop a whole picture of him/herself rather than just a picture of the autism spectrum. Working on a well produced document which gradually works through information and issues over time tends to be the most effective approach.

Some students who are ready for this information can find it helpful and it provides reasons and answers for some of the attributes they have noticed about themselves but did not have a prior understanding of.

Suggestions for helping children with autism to learn

CONCLUDING COMMENTS

This chapter has considered a few of the many questions that teachers and TAs have about individual children they work with and about issues about the autism spectrum in general. As stated earlier, there are no definite answers. The replies rather serve to encourage further thinking about the question areas and share some ideas that teachers and teaching assistants have effectively drawn upon to problem solve.

FURTHER READING

- Plimley, L., Bowen, M. and Morgan, H. (2007) *Autistic Spectrum Disorders in the Early Years*. London: Paul Chapman.
- Plimley, L. and Bowen, M. (2006) *Autistic Spectrum Disorders in the Secondary School*. London: Paul Chapman.

Useful Web Sites

www.widgit.com Provides information on what symbols do and how they provide a visual support to children with more complex needs. Also provides information on current widgit software for producing symbols.

www.symbolworld.org Provides examples of how symbols can be used to support stories, news, life skills sequencing pictures, etc.

www.do2learn.com Provides games, e.g. emotions, numeracy, etc., which are easily accessible for using with pupils. The site also provides some resources on organization tools that can be downloaded and printed off where appropriate, e.g. maths helpers, calendars, etc.

www.childrenwithspecialneeds.com Click into downloads for a range of photograph pictures, icons, on topics like food, clothes, menus, toys, etc.

www.visualstrategies.com Linda Hogdon has written a range of excellent visual strategies books and has some useful picture downloads. You can join her e-mail newsletter list for updates.

www.TEACCH.com The TEACCH web site provides information on the TEACCH approach and on a range of research as well as information on useful materials such as the Tasks Galore books, which provide a range of visually structured tasks which are useful in a variety of school contexts.

www.shoeboxtasks.com You can view and order shoebox self-contained tasks, which provide a range of different level activities, particularly for children with autism and learning difficulties.

www.preschoolfun.com Click on the thumbnail sketches and see a range of activities which give ideas about tasks which have been structured for young children on the autism spectrum to use.

www.pecs.org.uk Picture Exchange Communication Systems are used successfully with pupils in a variety special school and other school settings.

www.nas.org.uk The National Autistic Society web site provides some very easy-to-read and useful downloadable information on autism, Asperger's syndrome and associated topics.

Bibliography

Atwood, T. (1998) *Asperger's Syndrome. A guide for parents and professionals.* London: Jessica Kingsley.

Cumine, V., Leach, J. and Stevenson, G. (1998) *Asperger Syndrome. A Practical Guide for Teachers.* London: David Fulton.

Cumine, V., Leach, J. and Stevenson, G. (2000) *Autism in the Early Years.* London: David Fulton.

Dunn Buron, K. and Curis, M. (2003) *The Incredible Five-point Scale. Assisting Students with Autism Spectrum Disorders in understanding Social Interactions and controlling their Emotional Responses.* Shawnee Mission, KS: Autism Asperger Publishing.

Eckenrode, L., Fennell, P. and Hearsey, K. (2004a) *Tasks Galore Early Education.* Raleigh, NC: Tasks Galore Publishing.

Eckenrode, L., Fennell, P. and Hearsey, K. (2004b) *Tasks Galore for the Real World.* Raleigh, NC: Tasks Galore Publishing.

Eckenrode, L., Fennell, P. and Hearsey, K. (2005) *Tasks Galore Making Groups Meaningful.* Raleigh, NC: Tasks Galore Publishing

Faherty, C. (2000) *Asperger's. What does it mean to me?* Arlington, TX: Future Horizons.

Gagnon, E. (2006) *Power Cards. Using Special Interests to Motivate Children and Youth with Asperger Syndrome and Autism.* Shawnee Mission, KS: Autism Asperger Publishing.

Grandin, T. (1995) *Thinking in Pictures and other Reports from my Life with Autism.* New York: Doubleday.

Gray, C. (2000) *The New Social Story Book*, illustrated edition. Arlington, TX: Future Horizons.

Gray, C. and Leigh-White, A. (2002) *My Social Stories Book.* London: Jessica Kingsley.

Hodgdon, L. (1999) *Solving Behaviour Problems in Autism. Improving Communication with Visual Strategies.* Troy, MI: Quirk Roberts.

Ling, J. (2006) *I can't do that. My Social Stories to help with Communication, Self-care and Personal Skills.* London: Paul Chapman.

Mesibov, G. and Howley, M. (2003) *Accessing the Curriculum for Pupils with Autistic Spectrum Disorders. Using the TEACCH Programme to help Inclusion*. London: David Fulton.

Mesibov, G., Shea, V. and Schopler, E. (2004) *The TEACCH Approach to Autism Spectrum Disorders*. New York: Springer.

Plimley, L. and Bowen, M. (2006a) *Supporting Pupils with Autistic Spectrum Disorders. A Guide for School Support Staff*. London: Paul Chapman.

Plimley, L. and Bowen, M. (2006b) *Autistic Spectrum Disorders in the Secondary School*. London: Paul Chapman.

Plimley, L. and Bowen, M. (2007) *Social Skills and Autistic Spectrum Disorders*. London: Paul Chapman.

Plimley, L., Bowen, M. and Morgan, H. (2007) *Autistic Spectrum Disorders in the Early Years*. London: Paul Chapman.

Sainsbury, C. (2000) *Martian in the Playground*. Bristol: Lucky Duck Publications.

Shimmin, S. and White, H. (2006) *Every Day a Good Day. Establishing Routines in your Early Years Setting*. London: Paul Chapman.

Shore, S. (2003) *Beyond the Wall. Personal Experiences with Autism and Asperger Syndrome, second edition*. Shawnee Mission, KS: Autism Asperger Publishing.

Smith Myles, B., Trautman, M. L. and Schelvan, R. L. (2004) *The Hidden Curriculum. Practical Solutions for Understanding Unstated Rules in Social Situations*. Shawnee Mission, KS: Autism Asperger Publishing.

Wiley, L. (1999) *Pretending to be Normal. Living with Asperger's Syndrome*. London: Jessica Kingsley.

Whitaker, P. (2001) *Challenging Behaviour and Autism. Making Sense – making Progress. A Guide to Preventing and Managing Challenging Behaviour for Parents and Teachers*. London: National Autistic Society.

Wing, L. (1996) *The Autistic Spectrum*. London: Constable.

Index